CLINICAL, GENETIC AND MOLECULAR PRECURSOR FEATURES IN COLORECTAL NEOPLASIA

Clinical, Genetic and Molecular Precursor Features in Colorectal Neoplasia

Kjetil Søreide
and
Håvard Søiland

Nova Science Publishers, Inc.
New York

Copyright © 2008 by Nova Science Publishers, Inc.

All rights reserved. No part of this book may be reproduced, stored in a retrieval system or transmitted in any form or by any means: electronic, electrostatic, magnetic, tape, mechanical photocopying, recording or otherwise without the written permission of the Publisher.

For permission to use material from this book please contact us:
Telephone 631-231-7269; Fax 631-231-8175
Web Site: http://www.novapublishers.com

NOTICE TO THE READER

The Publisher has taken reasonable care in the preparation of this book, but makes no expressed or implied warranty of any kind and assumes no responsibility for any errors or omissions. No liability is assumed for incidental or consequential damages in connection with or arising out of information contained in this book. The Publisher shall not be liable for any special, consequential, or exemplary damages resulting, in whole or in part, from the readers' use of, or reliance upon, this material.

Independent verification should be sought for any data, advice or recommendations contained in this book. In addition, no responsibility is assumed by the publisher for any injury and/or damage to persons or property arising from any methods, products, instructions, ideas or otherwise contained in this publication.

This publication is designed to provide accurate and authoritative information with regard to the subject matter covered herein. It is sold with the clear understanding that the Publisher is not engaged in rendering legal or any other professional services. If legal or any other expert assistance is required, the services of a competent person should be sought. FROM A DECLARATION OF PARTICIPANTS JOINTLY ADOPTED BY A COMMITTEE OF THE AMERICAN BAR ASSOCIATION AND A COMMITTEE OF PUBLISHERS.

LIBRARY OF CONGRESS CATALOGING-IN-PUBLICATION DATA

Clinical, genetic, and molecular precursor features in colorectal neoplasia / Kjetil Søreide, Håvard Søiland, editors.
   p. ; cm.
 Includes bibliographical references and index.
 ISBN 978-1-60456-714-4 (softcover)
 1. Colon (Anatomy)--Cancer--Genetic aspects. 2. Rectum--Cancer--Genetic aspects. 3. Colon (Anatomy)--Cancer--Molecular aspects. 4. Rectum--Cancer--Molecular aspects. I. Søreide, Kjetil. II. Søiland, Håvard.
 [DNLM: 1. Colorectal Neoplasms--prevention & control. 2. Early Diagnosis. 3. Precancerous Conditions--diagnosis. 4. Precancerous Conditions--genetics. WI 529 C641 2008]
RC280.C6C57   2008
616.99'4347042--dc22   2008016273

Published by Nova Science Publishers, Inc. ✣ *New York*

Contents

Preface		**vii**
Chapter 1	Introduction	**1**
Chapter 2	Colorectal Carcinogenesis	**3**
Chapter 3	Hereditary Colorectal Cancers	**7**
Chapter 4	Inflammation and Colorectal Cancer	**15**
Chapter 5	Early Colorectal Cancer	**21**
Chapter 6	Microsatellite Instability	**33**
Chapter 7	Epigenetic Silencing	**45**
Chapter 8	Cyclooxygenase-2 and Colorectal Neoplasia	**49**
Chapter 9	Trypsin in Colorectal Cancer	**55**
Chapter 10	Other Proteinase-Systems	**59**
Chapter 11	Conclusions	**65**
References		**67**
Index		**99**

PREFACE

The understanding of the mechanisms that explain the initiation and early evolution of colorectal cancer is evolving. This should facilitate the development of new approaches to effective prevention and intervention. Over the past years, deficiencies in the current adenoma-carcinoma model for colorectal cancer, in which APC mutation is placed at the point of initiation, have been suggested. Several pathways through which cancer may develop seem to exist, such as 'chromosomal instability' (CIN), 'microsatellite instability' (MSI), and most recently the 'serrated pathway' involving epigenetic changes. Parallel to discoveries in molecular pathways are the increased awareness of early and precursor features of the colorectal mucosa detected and treated by endoscopic and minimal-invasive techniques. Thus, new staging and classification systems have been developed to guide the clinician in diagnosis and choice of treatment.

While most colorectal cancer develops sporadically (i.e. no known genetically defined risk) about 5-7% develop CRC on the basis of some hereditary syndrome. Lessons learned from the hereditary syndromes such as HNPCC and FAP have facilitated increased understanding of the basic molecular mechanisms of cancer development. For example, MSI causes hereditary non-polyposis colorectal cancer (HNPCC), and occurs as an important pathway in about 15-20% of sporadic colorectal cancers. Serrated adenomas of the colorectum show features intermediate between hyperplastic polyps and adenomas, and serve as a prototype for understanding of epigenetic mechanisms. Genes implicated in the regulation of apoptosis and DNA repair may underlie the early development of colorectal cancer. Inactivation of these genes may occur not by mutation or loss but through epigenetic silencing mediated by methylation of the gene's promoter region. MLH1 and MGMT are examples of DNA repair genes that are silenced by methylation. The "serrated" pathway of neoplasia is driven by inhibition of apoptosis and the subsequent inactivation of DNA repair genes by promoter methylation. The earliest lesions in this pathway are aberrant crypt foci (ACF). These may develop into hyperplastic polyps or transform while still of microscopic size into admixed polyps, serrated adenomas, or traditional adenomas. Although the basic mechanisms are not yet clear, there is increased understanding of the clinicopathological consequences. The genetic mechanisms differ in hereditary (germline mutation) and sporadic (epigenetic silencing) colorectal cancers.

Protease-systems are activated in early precursor stages in colorectal neoplasia, and contribute to proliferation, invasion, and metastasis. The interactions of extracellular matrix, stroma cells, and the immune cells on tumor cells have gained increasing interest over the past years. As a key-link in this aspects serves the cyclooxygenases (COX) and prostaglandines involved in inflammation – but also in cell proliferation and invasive and metastatic mechanisms – and amenable to inhibition by NSAIDs and coxibs. Better understanding of the tumor 'neighborhood' may give way for new preventive, prognostic, predictive and therapeutic factors.

Obviously, complete coverage of all aspects of colorectal cancerogenesis is an extensive endeavor. Thus, this book sets focus on selected clinical and molecular aspects of colorectal precursor lesions; from the endoscopically detected colorectal polyp, major molecular mechanisms, and aspects of protease-systems in colorectal cancer development.

Future research on colorectal cancer needs to be stratified according to the appropriate clinical features and their associated genetic pathways involved in order to further explore important molecular mechanisms and clinicopathological consequences of chromosomal, microsatellite and epigenetic mechanisms.

Chapter 1

INTRODUCTION

Every year, nearly one million people worldwide develop colorectal cancer (CRC), of whom about 50% are expected to die within 5 years[1-3]. CRC develops either sporadically (85%), as part of a hereditary cancer syndrome (<10%), or on a background of inflammatory bowel disease. Traditionally, it has been believed that the adenoma-carcinoma sequence underlies development of CRC in most patients, from which two distinct pathways have been identified – the *microsatellite instability (MSI)* and the *chromosomal instability (CIN)* pathways [4-9]. Discovery of these two pathways has led to the paradigm of CRC as a genetically heterogeneous disease [5, 8, 10]. Characterized by different clinical outcomes CRC with MSI has a better prognosis compared with stage-matched microsatellite stable cancers [11-15]. Genomic and transcriptomic differences exist between microsatellite unstable and stable CRC. Some of these differences may be used as diagnostic, predictive or prognostic markers [4, 13, 16-19]. Furthermore, current evidence suggest the additional inclusion of a third pathway; the *serrated adenoma* pathway – this involves epigenetic mechanisms which have just recently been discovered. Irrespective of these major mechanisms of carcinogenesis, the current years have seen growing interest in protease-related involvement in cancer, largely due to the possibility of therapeutic inhibition. Trypsin, protease-related receptors, and matrix metalloproteinases are but a few mentioned in this chapter [20]. Furthermore, clinical awareness of so-called *de novo* cancers, and improvements in endoscopic imaging and techniques has rendered new staging systems of early colorectal neoplasia and precancers for which some are mentioned in this chapter. As such, this chapter explores current knowledge about clinical aspects and molecular mechanisms in colorectal (pre)neoplasia and how they may foster new modes for early detection, prevention, and therapy.

Chapter 2

COLORECTAL CARCINOGENESIS

Development of CRC from an adenoma to carcinoma may take several decades. The risk of CRC begins to increase after the age of 40 years and rises sharply at the ages 50–55 years; the risk doubles with each succeeding decade, reaching a peak by age 75 years. Cancer as such, is the result of an accumulation of genetic alterations that allows growth of neoplastic cells with phenotypic hallmark characteristics: self-sufficiency in growth signals, insensitivity to anti-growth signals, evasion of apoptosis, limitless replicative potential, sustained angiogenesis, the ability to invade tissues and metastasise [20-22].

The multigene, clonal evolution, and selection model of initiation and progression of CRC proposed by Fearon & Vogelstein originally identified the *APC* gene, genes on *18q*, and the *K-ras* and *p53* genes as those in which mutations contribute to the evolution of CRC [23]. Although confirmed by later studies, many additional genes are also involved [23-28]. However, rather than representing a linear model of required accumulative mutations in the *APC*, *K-ras*, and *p53* genes (< 10% of all CRCs have all mutations) recent studies suggest they may each represent alternative, multiple mutational pathways in colorectal cancerogenesis [29], with specific associated chromosomal aberrations [30], and distinct clinical outcomes [31].

Nonetheless, knowledge derived from families with Familial Adenomatous Polyposis (FAP) or Hereditary Non-Polyposis Colorectal Cancer (HNPCC), helped establish the early model of colorectal carcinogenesis [23, 25]. Hereditary syndromes have germline mutations in specific genes (mutation in the tumor suppressor gene *APC* on chromosome *5q* in FAP; mutated DNA-mismatch repair genes in HNPCC) that greatly increase the lifetime risk for developing CRC (>80% in HNPCC) compared to the general population.

Sporadic CRC develops through randomly acquired somatic mutations in several of the same genes found in hereditary cancers. However, the rate of random mutational events alone cannot account for the number of genetic alterations found in most human cancers [32]. For this reason, it has been suggested that destabilization of the genome may be a prerequisite early in carcinogenesis [33]. This "mutator phenotype" is best understood in CRC, in which there are at least two separate destabilizing pathways (figure 1).

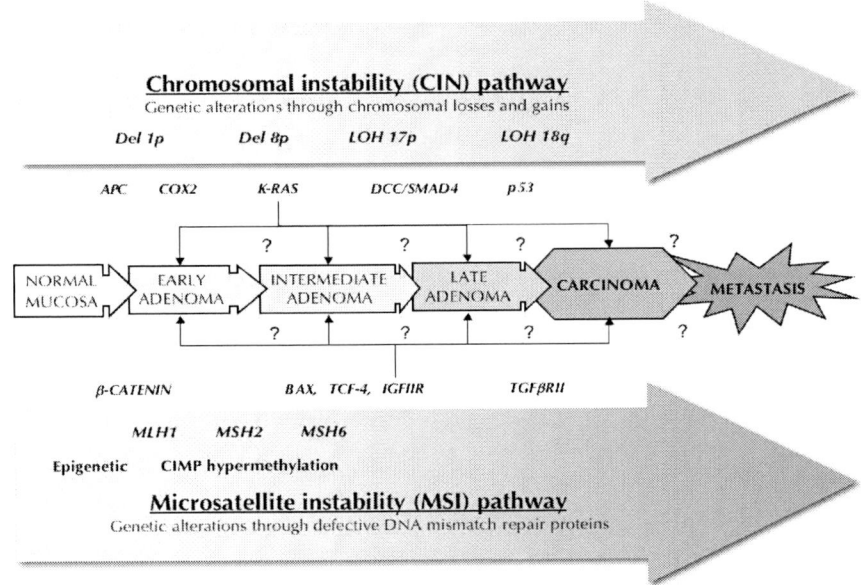

Legend: Characteristics of the major pathways in colorectal cancer. The adenoma-carcinoma sequence develops on the background of different types of genetic instability, including epigenetic silencing of important genes. Various genes seem to play a role according to their underlying pathway of development.

Abbreviations denotes: *APC, adenomatous polyposis coli*; *BAX, Bcl-2-associated X protein*; CIMP, CpG island methylator phenotype; *COX, cyclo-oxygenase*; *DCC, deleted in colorectal cancer*; *IGF-IIR, insulin-like growth factor II receptor*; LOH, loss of heterozygosity; *MLH, MutL homologue*; *MSH, MutB homologue*; *Smad, mothers against decapentaplegic homologue (Drosophila)*; *TCF, T cell factor*, *TGF-βR, transforming growth factor β receptor.*

The figure is derived from Søreide *et al*. Copyright British Journal of Surgery Society Ltd. Reproduced with permission. Permission is granted by John Wiley & Sons Ltd on behalf of the BJSS Ltd.

Figure 1. Major genetic instability pathways in colorectal cancer.

The most common genetic pathway (approximately 85% of CRCs) is characterized by allelic losses, chromosomal amplifications, and translocations [7-9, 25, 34-40]. Deletion at *1p* and *8p*, as well as *loss of heterozygosity* (LOH) of *17p* and *18q* are frequent in CRC. Such alterations are characteristic of the *chromosomal-instability pathway (CIN)*, also referred to as the microsatellite-stability pathway (MSS). The second pathway (involving about 15-20% of sporadic CRCs) is referred to as the *microsatellite-instability pathway (MSI)* [4]. Such tumours display frameshift mutations and base-pair substitutions that are commonly found in short, tandemly repeated nucleotide sequences known (i.e. CACACACA; CA_4) as microsatellites [27, 41-44]. This form of genetic destabilization is most commonly caused by loss of the DNA mismatch-repair function, as reviewed later in this chapter. Lastly, *epigenetic silencing*, the 'new-kid-on-the-block' in cancerogenesis, and proposed as the third pathway in CRC is enlightened and demonstrated further in the section on serrated adenomas. A plethora of molecular pathways exist in CRC development and progression. In this chapter, the focus will be set on some of the protease-related pathways found in both early and advanced CRC.

Chapter 3

HEREDITARY COLORECTAL CANCERS

Genetic alterations play a role in the development of all colorectal malignancies. In the majority of cases the mutations are spontaneous and not in the germline cells and, therefore, have no implications for the future generations (figure 2). However, as many as up to 30% of colorectal cancers have a potentially identifiable genetic (albeit not hereditary) cause [45, 46]. The specific genes responsible for most of the cases of moderate–risk CRC have yet to be characterized. However, in the high–risk (hereditary) cases many of the genes have been identified. These high–risk cases account for 3–5% of all colon cancers, these patients have a substantial life-time risk of colon cancer and includes familial adenomatous polyposis (FAP), hereditary non-polyposis colon cancer (HNPCC), and hamartomatous disorders; juvenile polyposis syndrome and Peutz–Jeghers syndrome. Early identification and intervention can significantly reduce the risk of malignancy in these patients.

The genetic colon cancer syndromes can be broadly classified in two categories – *presence* or *absence* of gastrointestinal polyps. Large numbers of polyps distinguishes the polyposis syndromes, which further can be classified histologically as either adenomatous or hamartomatous. There can also be polyps in the nonpolyposis syndromes but these are less numerous and more difficult to distinguish from sporadic adenomas. A brief delineation of the most important syndromes and their associated features are given.

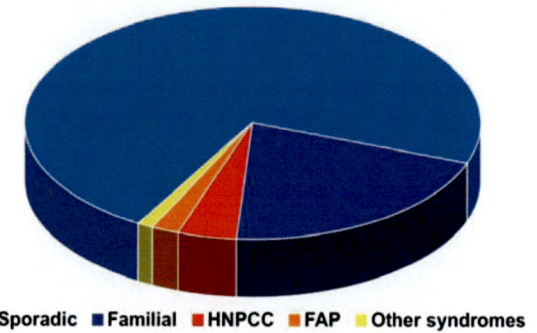

■ Sporadic ■ Familial ■ HNPCC ■ FAP ■ Other syndromes

Legend: While most CRC are sporadic (70-80%), about 10-20% are thought to have some kind of familial, unidentified genetic predisposition. Hereditary syndromes account for < 5-6% of all CRC, where HNPCC and FAP are the most frequently encountered.

Figure 2. Aetiologic distribution of CRC.

HEREDITARY NON-POLYPOSIS COLORECTAL CANCER (HNPCC)

In 1966, Henry Lynch described families without colonic polyposis who developed colon, endometrial and gastric cancer at early ages [47-49]. These cancer family syndromes were later named Lynch syndromes 1 and 2, and then eventually given its current designation as HNPCC. In the early 1990s it was recognized that the tumors occurring in patients with HNPCC had a characteristic molecular change called microsatellite instability, initially referred to as replication error (RER) [28, 50]. Shortly thereafter the genes responsible were found – the mismatch repair (MMR) genes [25, 27, 51].

At least 5 genes have been identified and have been implicated in HNPCC families or atypical HNPCC families. MSH2 on chromosome 2p, and MLH1 on chromosome 3p, account for the majority of genetically defined cases. From 15-60% have mutations in these genes. Other genes are PMS1, PMS2 and MSH6. Over 90% of all colorectal cancers in HNPCC patients demonstrate microsatellite instability.

HNPCC is the most common form of hereditary colorectal cancers, and account for 1-6% of all colorectal malignancies. The clinical features are families with clustering of HNPCC cancers; colorectal, gastric, endometrial, small bowel, renal and ureteral cancers, and onset of these cancers at a young age. It is inherited as an autosomal dominant decease, with 80% penetrance. The lifetime risk for cancer is 80% at 70 years of age. The mean age of colon cancer is around

45 years, which precedes the age of sporadic CRC by 20 years. Cancer can occur during adolescence, but it is unusual before the third decade of life.

Table 1. Features of HNPCC

Inheritance pattern	Autosomal dominant
Incidence	1:2000
Gene	Mismatch repair genes, 5 different genes
Colon polyps	Few or none
Lifetime CRC risk	80% risk at 70 years, mean age of CRC 44 years
Localisation	Most right-sided colon cancer, but also multiple (synchrone or metachrone)
Extra-colonic cancers	gastric, endometrial, small bowel, renal and ureteral cancers
Clinical	Amsterdam criteria 1 and 2, and Bethesda(se text and table)
Surveillance	Unclear, but full colonscopy from 20-25 years, every year or every other year. Endometrial cancer screening
Treatment	Depends on the localisation of the tumor, subtotal or total colectomy with close surveillance of the rest of the colon.

Table 2. Amsterdam criteria

Amsterdam I criteria

1. Three or more relatives with colorectal cancer, one whom is a first-degree relative of the other two;
2. Colorectal cancer involving at least two generations.
3. One or more colorectal cancers diagnosed at age <50 years.

Amsterdam II criteria

1. Three or more relatives with a HNPCC-associated cancer (colorectal, endometrial, small bowel, ureter, renal pelvis), one of whom is a first-degree relative of the other two.
2. Colorectal cancer involving at least two generations.
3. One or more colorectal cancers diagnosed at age <50 years.

Modified Amsterdam criteria

1. Very small families which cannot be further expanded can be considered as HNPCC with only two colorectal cancers in first-degree relatives; colorectal cancers must involve at least two generations, and at least one colorectal cancer must be diagnosed at age < 55 years.
2. In families with two first-degree relatives affected by colorectal cancer, the presence of a third relative with an unusual early-onset neoplasm or endometrial cancer is sufficient.

Table 3. Bethesda criteria

Bethesda criteria

1. Amsterdam criteria
2. Two HNPCC-related cancers, including synchronous and metachronous colorectal cancers or associated extracolonic cancers
3. Colorectal cancer and a first-degree relative with colorectal cancer and / or a HNPCC-related extracolonic cancer and / or a colorectal adenoma; one of the cancers diagnosed at age < 45 years, and the adenoma diagnosed age < 40 years
4. Colorectal cancer or endometrial cancer diagnosed at age <45 years
5. Right-sided colorectal cancer with an undifferentiated pattern on histology diagnosed at age < 45 years
6. Signet-ring cell-type colorectal cancer diagnosed at age < 45 years
7. Adenomas diagnosed at age < 40 years

Revised Bethesda criteria

1. Colorectal cancer diagnosed at age < 50 years
2. Synchronous or metachrounus colorectal or other HNPCC-associated tumors regardless of age.
3. Colorectal cancer diagnosed at age < 60 years with histologic findings of infiltrating lymphocytes, Crohn`s-like lymphocytic reaction, mucinous/signet ring differentiation or medullary growth pattern.
4. Colorectal cancer in one or more first-degree relative(s) with an HNPCC-related tumor, with one of the cancers being diagnosed at age 50 years.
5. Colorectal cancer diagnosed in two or more first or second-degree relatives with HNPCC-related tumors, regardless of age.

The diagnostic criteria for HNPCC continue to evolve (table 2 and 3). The Amsterdam criteria were developed in 1990 for research purposes. Initially, the criteria were not intended for diagnostic purposes and were exclusively for clinical work. Thus, these criteria have later been revised (Amsterdam 2 and the modified Amsterdam; table 2) [49]. The Bethesda criteria were developed to identify patients who would benefit from microsatellite instability testing (table 3), and also these have been revised and simplified [52, 53]. The current diagnostic criteria and algorithms for screening of HNPCC continue to evolve [48, 54-58].

FAMILIAL ADENOMATOUS POLYPOSIS (FAP)

FAP was the first polyposis syndrome to be recognized and remains the most characterized (table 4). FAP is a highly penetrant autosomal–dominant disorder caused by a mutation in the APC gene, located on chromosome 5q21. APC is a tumor suppressor gene, and besides being the cause of FAP is also involved in the early initiation of sporadic CRC [59-61]. Inactivation of the gene product constitutes the initial development of CRC. Over 700 different decease-causing APC mutations have been reported to date. By routine screening methods, as many as 20-30% of classical FAP patients have no detectable APC mutation. However, on mono–allelic mutation analysis, more than 95% of FAP patients will have an identifiable mutation.

Table 4. Features of FAP

Inheritance pattern	Autosomal dominant, but one third is new spontaneous mutations
Incidence	1:10000–1:18000
Gene	Mutation in the adenomatous polyposis coli gene (APC), almost 100% penetrance
Colon polyps	Hundreds to thousands of adenomatous polyps in the whole colon and rectum, often arise in the teens
Lifetime CRC risk	Nearly 100% at age 35-40 years
Localisation	70-80% occur on the left side
Extra-colonic cancers	Small bowel cancer, Desmoid tumors, periampullary cancers, thyroid cancers
Clinical	Amsterdam criteria 1 and 2, and Bethesda(se text and table)
Surveillance	Endoscopy surveillance probably from puberty or from onset of symptoms.
Treatment	Studies suggest benefit from COX-inhibitors. Proctocolectomy recommended for all patients probably during adolescence, excellent for colon cancers, but prevention of extracolonic malignancies remains challenging.

In northern Europe it is estimated roughly 1 in 13,000 to 1 in 18,000 live births will have FAP. The hallmark of FAP is the development of hundreds to thousands of adenomatous polyps in the colon and rectum, usually starting in adolescence, and almost every patient will get a progression to CRC by the age of 40 years – significantly younger than sporadic cancers. As many as 70-80% of the tumors occur in the left–sided large bowel – which contrasts the HNPCC cancers which tend to occur in the right colon. Only a small fraction of CRC is caused by FAP (<1%) and this fraction is decreasing with improved diagnostics and treatment.

Upper gastrointestinal polyps are present in nearly 90% of FAP patients by the age of 70 years. Small bowel cancer is the third leading cause of death in FAP patients (8%), apart from metastatic CRC (58%) and desmoid tumours (10%). One retrospective Swedish study found among 180 FAP patients a cumulative risk of periampullary adenocarcinoma of 10% by the age of 60 yr. There are some variants of the FAP syndrome:

Attenuated FAP

These patients develop fewer polyps than the FAP patients, and at a later age (third decade). The polyps tend to be more proximally and the risk of colon cancer is slightly lower. These patients often have no family history of CRC and extra–colonic features are much more rare (table 5).

Table 5. Attenuated FAP

Inheritance pattern	Autosomal dominant
Incidence	1:8000
Gene	APC gene mutation; in the extreme proximal or distal portion of the gene
Colon polyps	Fewer than 100 adenomas, and predominantly proximal
Lifetime CRC risk	Up to 70% at 80 year
Localisation	Most right-sided colon cancer
Extra-colonic cancers	Seldom
Clinical	Amsterdam criteria 1 and 2, and Bethesda(se text and table)
Surveillance	Endoscopy surveillance
Treatment	Colectomy when the polyps become numerous or dysplastic.

MYH Associated Polyposis

These patients have the phenotype like attenuated FAP patients, but have no mutation in the FAP gene, and they have no family history of CRC. It is inherited in in an autosomal recessive pattern, and they have a mutation in the MYH gene. MYH, located on the short arm of chromosome 1, is a base excision repair gene preventing mutations from product of oxidative damage. There is a low spontaneous mutation rate, and the penetrance is high. It involves a possible 50% increased risk of CRC. There are but a few studies on this entity, so the natural history of the patients are not well known.

HAMARTOMATOUS POLYPOSIS SYNDROMES

The hamartomatous polyposis syndromes account for less than 1% of CRC. To date, there are 7 inherited hamartomatous polyposis syndrome described; Peutz–Jeghers syndrome, juvenile polyposis syndrome, Cowden's disease (which is associated with mutation in the tumor suppressor PTEN), Bannayan-Ruvalcaba-

Riley syndrome, basal cell nevus syndrome, neurofibromatosis 1, and multiple endocrine neoplasia syndrome 2B. The newly identified mixed polyposis syndrome is a variant of juvenile polyposis, but have both adenomatous and hamartomatous polyps.

All these syndromes are inherited in an autosomal dominant fashion. The two most common syndromes are the Peutz–Jeghers syndrome and the juvenile polyposis syndrome.

Peutz-Jeghers Syndrome (PJS)

The typical feature of PJS is childhood onset of polyps and some typical mucocutaneous pigmentation (table 6). PJS is caused by a gene named LKB1, which is a serine–threonine kinase located on chromosome 19p. The LKB1 is thought to function as a tumor suppressor gene. About 50-75% of the patients have this mutation.

Table 6. Peutz-Jeghers syndrome (PJS)

Inheritance pattern	Autosomal dominant with high penetrance
Incidence	1:10000-1/100000
Gene	Mutation in the LKB1 gene, a tumor suppressor gene, found in 50-75% of the patients
Colon polyps	Multiple hamartomatous polyps in the whole gastrointestinal tract, most in the small intestine.
Lifetime CRC risk	50-90% of the patient will develop cancer, and 40% of this is CRC.
Localisation	Entire colon
Extra-colonic cancers	Stomach, esophagus, small intestine, and pancreas cancer. They have also increased risk for breast, ovarian, cervical, thyroid, lung and prostate cancers
Clinical	Multiple mucocutane pigmentation in the first year of living (perioral and oral mucosa, face, forearms palms, soles, fingers and perianal area)
Surveillance	Annual or biannual endoscopy, small bowel studies, ultrasound of ovaries and mammogram
Treatment	According to pathology.

PJS patients develop multiple black or brown macules on the oral mucosa, in the face, and on the distal extremities. They commonly occur on the lips and it often appears in the first year of living. The polyps are in the whole gastrointestinal tract, but mostly in the small intestine. Cancer develops in 50-90%

of the patients, with colon as the most usual site (40%), but also in stomach, esophagus, small intestine, pancreas, breast, ovarian, thyroid, prostate and lung.

Juvenile Polyposis

Juvenile polyposis is a very uncommon finding (table 7). These patients have multiple polyps in the gastrointestinal tract, and they often have other congenital abnormalities, like cardiac, craniofacial and bowel rotation. The exact cancer risk is unknown, but it is reported increased risk of colon, gastric, duodenal and pancreatic cancer.

Table 7. Juvenile polyposis

Inheritance pattern	Autosomal dominant
Incidence	1:100,000
Gene	Mutation in genes involved in the TGF-β signalling pathway have been implicated in some of the patients.
Colon polyps	At least threee juvenile polyps, but hundreds may develop over time throughout the gastrointestinal tract, Most polyps are in the colon and rectum
Lifetime CRC risk	Increased risk of cancer, CRC most frequently reported. Overall cancer risk may exceed 50%, in one study 68% at age 60 years, in another 21% developed CRC with a mean age of 34 years.
Localisation	-
Extra-colonic cancers	but also gastric, duodenal and pancreatic cancers are seen.
Clinical	often other congenital abnormalities (cardiac, craniofacial and bowel rotation).
Surveillance	Endoscopy with polypectomy from twelve years age
Treatment	if polyps are numerous or large; colectomy. The choice of surgical procedure is controversial

Chapter 4

INFLAMMATION AND COLORECTAL CANCER

INFLAMMATION AND CANCER

Tumors are complex tissues composed of ever-evolving neoplastic cells, matrix proteins that provide structural support and sequester biologically active molecules, and a cellular–stromal component (figure 3). Reciprocal interactions between neoplastic cells, activated host cells and the dynamic microenvironment in which they live, enable tumor growth and dissemination. It has become evident that early and persistent inflammatory responses observed in or around developing neoplasia regulates many aspects of tumor development (matrix remodelling, angiogenesis, malignant potential) by providing diverse mediators implicated in maintaining tissue homeostasis, e.g., soluble growth and survival factors, matrix remodelling enzymes, reactive oxygen species and a number of other bioactive molecules [62-65].

In 1863, Virchow hypothesized that malignant neoplasms occurred at sites of chronic inflammation [66]. Virchow reasoned that various "irritants" caused tissue injury, inflammation, and increased cell proliferation. Inflammation involves a complex reaction to microbial, chemical, or physical agents in vascularized tissue resulting in the influx of circulating leukocytes, connective tissue cells, and extracellular constituents consisting of fibrous proteins (collagen, elastin) and glycoproteins (fibronectin, laminin, and proteoglycans). Chronic inflammation may develop from unresolved symptomatic acute inflammation or may evolve insidiously over a period of months without apparent acute onset of clinical manifestations. Histopathologic features of chronic inflammation include the predominance of macrophages and lymphocytes, proliferation of nurturing structurally heterogeneous and hyperpermeable small blood vessels, fibrosis, and necrosis. Activated macrophages and lymphocytes are interactive in releasing inflammatory mediators or cytokines that amplify immune reactivity. Cytokines represent a family of biologic response modifiers including interleukins, chemokines, interferons, growth factors, and leukocyte colony-stimulating factors. The cytokines are secreted by leukocytes, connective tissue cells, and endothelial cells. Chemokines are proteins that stimulate leukocyte recruitment and migration as part of the host response to antigenic insults. In chronic inflammation, the protracted inflammatory response is often accompanied simultaneously by tissue destruction and repair.

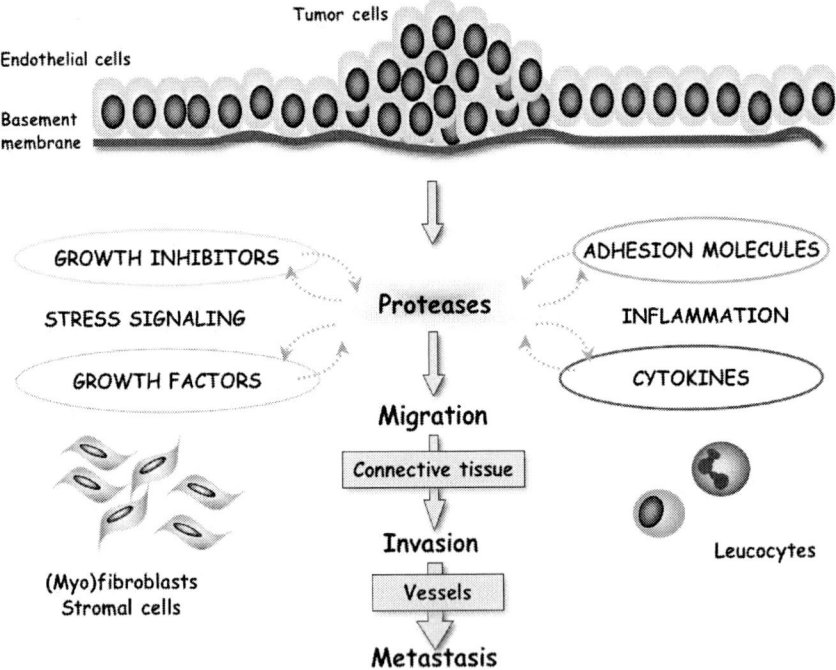

Legend: Tumorcells are influenced by a number of factors promoting cell proliferation, migration, invasion, and metastasis. The extracellular matrix (ECM) and inflammatory systems contribute via direct and indirect influences and mediators.

Figure 3. Tumor microenvironment.

Dvorak [67] noted similarities and differences between physiologic wound healing and mechanisms involved in the pathologic generation of supporting connective tissue (stroma) that sustains neoplastic cell proliferation and invasion. Dvorak referred to tumors as "*wounds that do not heal*" [67]. The infiltration of leukocytes in neoplastic tissue may be viewed as an antitumor response; however, there is compelling evidence that the infiltrate of activated macrophages and lymphocytes recruited from the microcirculation is a major source of proinflammatory cytokines, growth factors, and angiogenic factors. The extent of the leukocyte infiltration in solid tumors is controlled in part by the local production of chemokines by both neoplastic cells and stromal cells. The network of cytokines, chemokines, and growth factors interact with specific cell surface receptors that signal target genes involved in cell proliferation and influence tumor cell survival, neoangiogenesis, and migration of tumor cells into the stromal matrix (figure 3). Of interest is the recent finding that high levels of infiltrating memory T-cells (CD45RO+ cells) in the invasive front of CRCs, correlated with the absence of signs of early metastatic invasion of lymph or venous vessels, a less advanced pathological stage, and increased survival in patients with CRC [68].

Chronic inflammation and the metabolic products of phagocytosis are often accompanied by the excessive formation of reactive oxygen and nitrogen species that are potentially damaging to DNA, lipoproteins, and cell membranes. Inflammatory cells also release metabolites of arachidonic acid, or eicosanoids, including prostanoids or prostaglandins and leukotrienes [69-74]. The cyclo-oxygenases are key enzymes that control rate-limiting steps in prostaglandin synthesis and will be given further attention later in this chapter. The expression of the isoform COX-2 is induced by inflammatory and neoplastic cells, and metabolites produced by the action of COX-2 on arachidonic acid have been shown to impact various carcinogenic pathways. The neoplastic transformation of proliferating stem cells and subsequent tumor invasion may require a microenvironment of activated inflammatory cells and stromal cell elements.

INFLAMMATORY BOWEL DISEASE AND COLORECTAL CANCER

Inflammatory bowel disease (IBD) provides an excellent example of increased risk of neoplasia experienced by patients with chronic inflammation in gastrointestinal tissues [75]. Patients with ulcerative colitis (UC) and Crohn's disease (CD) are at increased risk for developing colorectal cancer [76-85]. To date, no known genetic basis has been identified to explain colorectal cancer predisposition in these inflammatory bowel diseases. Instead, it is assumed that chronic inflammation is what causes cancer. This is supported by the fact that colon cancer risk increases with longer duration of colitis, greater anatomic extent of colitis, the concomitant presence of other inflammatory manifestations such as primary sclerosing cholangitis, and the fact that certain drugs used to treat inflammation, such as 5-aminosalicylates and steroids, may prevent the development of colorectal cancer.

Ulceroinflammatory disease in UC is confined to the mucosa and submucosa and may extend throughout the rectum and colon; in approximately 10% of patients, the distal ileum may be involved (as so-called "backwash ileitis"). Crohn's disease (CD) is characterized by a *transmural* inflammatory process in the large or small intestine that exhibits mucosal damage, noncaseating granulomas, fissuring, and fistula formation. A classical feature of CD when multiple bowel segments are involved is the demonstration of "skip" lesions with intervening clinically normal bowel. The pathogenesis of IBD suggests that there has been an aberrant immune response to luminal indigenous microorganisms or ingested foreign antigens. The inflammatory response mediated by CD4+ T-cells is exaggerated, unregulated, and cytotoxic. The mucosal ulcerations would allow for microbial flora to gain access to submucosal lymphoid tissue and thus trigger an immune response.

RISK OF CANCER IN IBD

The risk of colorectal cancer in IBD patients increases with longer duration of disease and with extent of involvement of the large intestine [76]. In addition, the risk increases with the appearance and higher grade of dysplastic lesions. Dysplastic areas may appear flat or polypoid, localized, multifocal, or diffuse. The multicentricity of neoplasms commonly seen in IBD reflects "field cancerization" and suggests intraepithelial spread of preinvasive neoplastic cells or multiple clones of tumors. After an induction–latency interval of up to 10–15 years, the risk of cancer increases at the rate of 0.5% to 1% per year. In the study by Ekbom and colleagues [76], the incidence of colorectal cancer, as compared with the expected incidence, in the cohort was increased (standardized incidence ratio [ratio of observed to expected cases] = 5.7; 95% Confidence Interval: 4.6–7.0). They found that less extensive disease at diagnosis was associated with a lower risk; for patients with ulcerative proctitis, the standardized incidence ratio was 1.7

(95% CI: 0.8–3.2); for those with left-sided colitis, 2.8 (95% CI: 1.6–4.4); and for those with pancolitis (extensive colitis, or inflammation of the entire colon), 14.8 (95% CI: 11.4–18.9). Age at diagnosis and the extent of disease at diagnosis were strong and independent risk factors for colorectal cancer. For each increase in age group at diagnosis (less than 15 years, 15 to 29 years, 30 to 39 years, 40 to 49 years, 50 to 59 years, and greater than or equal to 60 years), the relative risk of colorectal cancer, adjusted for the extent of disease at diagnosis, decreased by about half (adjusted standardized incidence ratio = 0.51; 95% CI: 0.46–0.56). The absolute risk of colorectal cancer 35 years after diagnosis was 30% for patients with pancolitis at diagnosis and 40% for those given this diagnosis at less than 15 years of age. As such, colitis-associated colorectal cancer is diagnosed at a younger age than sporadic colorectal cancer in the general population. On microscopy, such cancers more often exhibit a mucinous or signet-ring cell histology. How these facts relate to genetic alterations remain unclear, but knowledge is evolving.

INFLAMMATORY MOLECULAR CARCINOGENESIS

The major carcinogenic pathways that lead to sporadic CRC, namely chromosomal instability, microsatellite instability, and hypermethylation, also occur in colitis-associated colorectal cancers. Unlike normal colonic mucosa, however, inflamed colonic mucosa demonstrates abnormalities in these molecular pathways even before any histological evidence of dysplasia or cancer. Whereas the reasons for this are unknown, oxidative stress likely plays a role. Reactive oxygen and nitrogen species produced by inflammatory cells can interact with key genes involved in carcinogenic pathways such as p53, DNA mismatch repair genes, and even DNA base excision-repair genes [86, 87]. Central players in inflammatory pathways, such as NF–κB and cyclo–oxygenases also contribute, as well as a number of inflammatory-regulated factors for which the evidence is evolving [74, 77, 88-96]. Administering agents that cause colitis in healthy rodents or genetically engineered cancer-prone mice accelerates the development of colorectal cancer. Mice genetically prone to inflammatory bowel disease also develop colorectal cancer especially in the presence of bacterial colonization.

IBD may be associated with manifestations of chronic inflammation and neoplasia in the biliary ductal system. An example of this is primary sclerosing cholangitis (PSC), which occurs in approximately 3% of patients with ulcerative colitis and less frequently (about 1%) in patients with Crohn disease. PSC is characterized by inflammation, cholestasis, and fibrosis in the intrahepatic and extrahepatic biliary ducts. The frequency of cholangiocarcinoma in patients with PSC has been estimated to vary between 5% and 20%. Manifestations of UC may be evident in 70% of PSC patients. The clinical course in PSC is not affected by medical or surgical treatment of IBD, suggesting common susceptibility and pathogenic factors rather than that IBD is a direct cause of PSC.

CANCER SURVEILLANCE IN IBD

Proposed guidelines for surveillance of patients with IBD aim to detect asymptomatic CRC [97, 98]. However, according to a recent Cochrane review [99] there is no clear evidence that surveillance colonoscopy prolongs survival in patients with extensive colitis. There is evidence that cancers tend to be detected at an earlier stage in patients who are undergoing surveillance, and these patients have a correspondingly better prognosis, but lead-time bias could contribute substantially to this apparent benefit. There is indirect evidence that surveillance is likely to be effective at reducing the risk of death from IBD-associated colorectal cancer and indirect evidence that it may be acceptably cost-effective [99]. However, as found in two recent studies, there was no apparent increased risk of CRC in those with UC as to the general North American population, and surveillance detected two thirds of the developing cancers in the IBD population under colonoscopic surveillance [100-102]. Thus, the debate will continue to evolve in the future as to the perceived risks and best clinical strategies for patients with IBD.

Chapter 5

EARLY COLORECTAL CANCER

The prognosis of CRC in the individual patient depends on the stage of the disease at the time of diagnosis. As a consequence, screening for CRC has been accepted in several countries, aiming at the diagnosis and treatment of premalign changes in the mucosa as well as to find asymptomatic invasive cancer [103, 104]. While faecal occult blood test (FOBT) has been demonstrated to be able to save lives in CRC screening [105-111], recent methods have focused on colonoscopy and the potential for detecting genetic alterations in stool [106, 112-114]. The traditional understanding of developing CRC is based on the concept of adenoma-carcinoma sequence [23, 25, 115-117]. According to this theory, benign adenomas of the colorectal mucosa gradually transform to invasive cancer over time, and thus, removal of an adenoma might prevent cancer. However, according to some reports, between 20-40% of all tumours may evolve from the colorectal mucosa *de novo* and grow invasively into the bowel wall [118-120]. Adenomatous remnants in invasive cancer have been found only in about 20% of the tumours [120, 121]. While the concept of *de novo* carcinogenesis was considered as a phenomenon related to Asian populations, it has gained more attention in the Western world during the past decade [115, 122].

As such, definition of neoplasia in the colorectal mucosa remains a central issue. According to the WHO classification [123], intramucosal neoplastic lesions are confined to the mucosal layer (i.e. mucosa, lamina propria and muscularis mucosae), and are graded to the degree of dysplasia (i.e. mild, moderate or high grade; low–grade or high–grade intraepithelial neoplasia). Invasive cancer is defined as tumour invading beyond the muscularis mucosae layer into the submucosa. However, Japanese pathologists consider intramucosal lesions as early colorectal cancer based on other features than solely invasion like nuclear and structural changes, thus possibly leading to higher incidence figures of early malignant lesion in the colorectum [124]. Accordingly, intramucosal lesions with high-grade dysplasia as defined by WHO may be diagnosed as intramucosal cancer according to the Japanese criteria. However, there has recently been achieved an international consensus with regard to classification of gastrointestinal epithelial neoplasia [125].

THE ABERRANT CRYPT FOCI (ACF)

The suggested first and earliest identifiable neoplastic lesions in the carcinogenetic model of the colon and rectum are so-called aberrant crypt foci (ACF) [126-130]. They are defined as small circumscript areas in the colorectal mucosa with enlarged crypts as compared to surrounding normal mucosa. It is thought that in the course of subsequent accumulation of biochemical and mutational changes some of the ACF develop to cancer.

The progression of ACF to polyp and, subsequently, to cancer parallels the accumulation of several molecular alterations and mutations whereby a small fraction of ACF evolve to CRC. Recent data indicate that, not uncommonly, some ACF bypass the polyp stage in their carcinogenesis thus reinforcing the importance of their early detection and our understanding of their pathogenesis. Since ACF were first detected in carcinogen-treated mice, research efforts have focused on these microscopically visible lesions both in animal and human models [127, 128, 131]. ACF show variable histological features [132], and can be grouped into differing categories by in vivo examination with high-magnification-chromoscopic-colonoscopy (HMCC). As expected, ACF are more frequently detected in distal animal and human colons coinciding with the geographic distribution of CRC. Various proteomic markers may be altered within ACF suggesting possible prospective pathological changes. These protein markers include calreticulin, transgelin, serotransferrin, triphosphate isomerase and carbonic anhydrase II [130]. Other markers of importance include carcinoembryonic antigen (CEA), β-catenin, placental cadherin (P-cadherin), epithelial cadherin (E-cadherin), inducible nitric oxide synthase (iNOS), cyclooxygenase (COX-2) and $p16^{INK4a}$. Genetic mutations of K-ras, B-raf, APC and p53 have been demonstrated in ACF as well as the epigenetic alterations of CpG island methylation [131, 133, 134]. Genomic instabilities (GI), illustrated by a higher GI index, microsatellite instability, loss of heterozygosity (LOH) and defects in mismatch repair (MMR) systems, are also expressed [126, 127, 129-131, 134]. These transformations may lead to the identification of the earliest pathological features initiating colon tumorigenesis [8, 130, 135, 136]. The long line of evidence developed over the past decade suggest that ACF might be an important, yet unresolved, biomarker for CRC [126-129, 134, 137].

COLORECTAL POLYPS

The incidence of colorectal adenomas has been estimated in a population based study at 3.7/100.000 [138], and polyps are found in up to 10% of asymptomatic persons undergoing sigmoidoscopy, and as many as 25% of those undergoing colonoscopy [139]. However, the true incidence rate is hard to be known exactly, as it depends strongly on the definition used for diagnosis and selection criteria of the population to be studied.

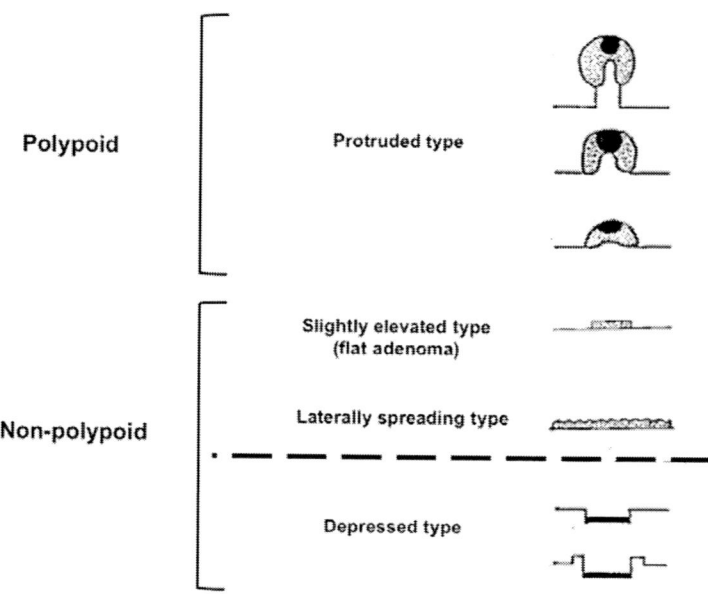

Figure 4. The Japanese Research Society classification of polyps.

Colorectal neoplasia research has traditionally focused on exophytically growing (protruding) tumours. However, during the past decades, Japanese researchers emphasised the importance of intramucosal premalignant and malign lesions with endophytical growth pattern and early invasion into the bowel wall.

The first case of depressed neoplastic lesions was reported by Kariya three decades ago [140]. Current concepts include both protruding, flat and depressed neoplastic lesions (figure 4) [141].

CLASSIFICATION OF NEOPLASTIC LESIONS

Haggit [142] introduced in 1985 a classification for protruding tumours in the colon and rectum (figure 5). The level of invasion into the polyp was shown to correlate well with prognosis, and is thus considered an important guideline in the treatment of this type of neoplasia.

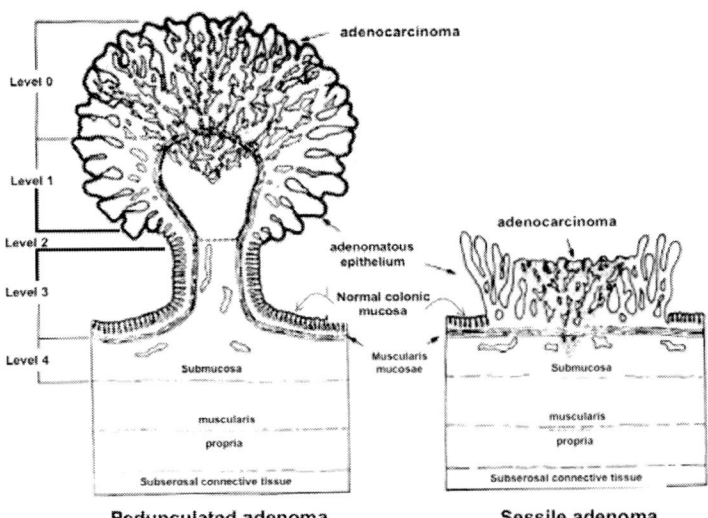

Legend:.
Level 0:   adenoma with intramucosal carcinoma (in situ).
Level 1:   penetration of malignant glands through the muscularis mucosa into the submucosa, within the polyp head.
Level 2:   the same submucosal invasion, but present at the junction of the head to the stalk.
Level 3:   invasion of the stalk.
Level 4:   invasion of the stalk's base at the connection to the colonic wall (this level corresponds to stage Dukes A).

Figure 5. Classification according to Haggitt. figure reprinted from GASTROENTEROLOGY, 89(2):328-336, Haggitt RC, et al. © 1985 American Gastroenterological Association

Non-protruding lesions are divided into flush/slightly elevated lesions, laterally spreading and depressed lesions [143]. It is important to notice that the various non-protruding lesions have varying potential with regard to invasion into the submucosa. While flat adenomas have mostly benign characteristica, depressed type lesions are considered more aggressive [144]. There is a sharp transition from malignant cells in the depressed lesion to the normal surrounding mucosa without adenomatous components [145]. This is considered as important support to the *de novo* carcinogenesis model in colorectal neoplasia. Furhtermore, the size of the neoplasia is of great prognostic importance. Kudo et al. [143] showed in a large number of colorectal neoplasias that depressed type lesions of 6-10 mm diameter showed submucosal invasion in about 24% as compared to 1.3% in protruding lesions and 0.5% in flush or slightly elevated lesions, and increased with the size of the lesion.

SUBMUCOSAL INVASION

Submucosal invasion is central in the understanding of early colorectal neoplasia. Classification of submucosal invasion is based on the division of the submucosa (sm) into three layers, from *sm1* to *sm3* (figure 6). Sm1 lesions are subdivided into three categories with regard to the degree of horizontal involvement of the upper submucosal layer (ratio of involving part and not-involving part). While sm1a + b lesions never metastasise, the malignant potential increases with deeper invasion into the submucosa [144]. Beside the depth of invasion, affection of submucosal vessels is also important. A strong relationship between submucosal invasion and potential of spread to regional lymph nodes and distant organs has been shown [143].

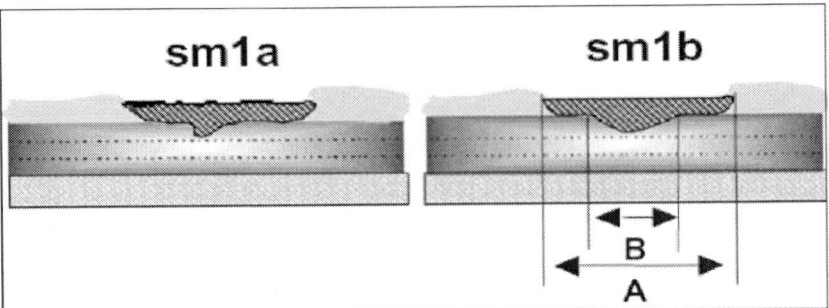
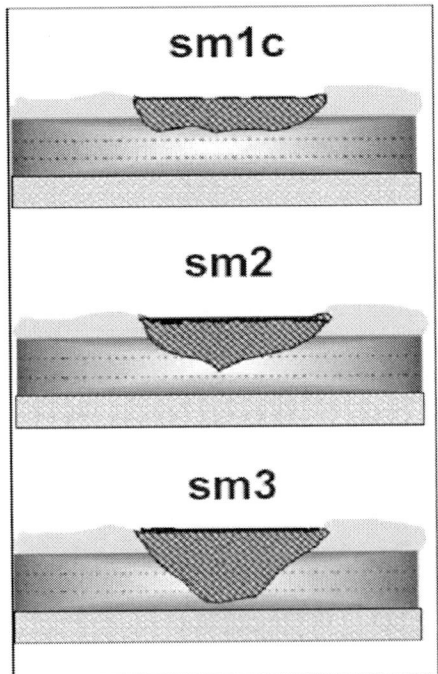

Legend: Degrees of submucosal invasion.
sm1: upper 1/3; sm1a: B/A ≤1/4; sm1b: B/A=1/4–1/2; sm1c: B/A ≥1/2.
sm2: middle 1/3.
sm3: lower 1/3.

Figure 6. Degrees of submucosal invasion.

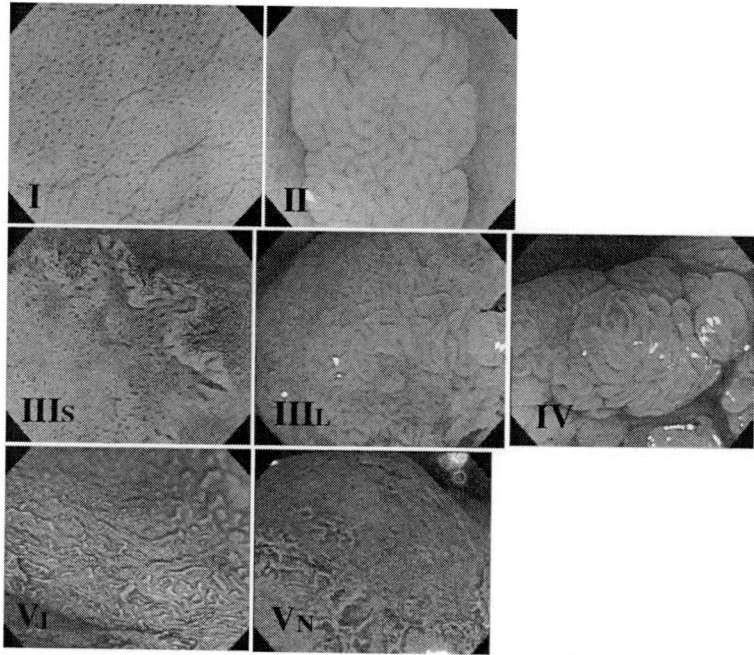

Legend: Classification of pit patterns: I, II, III$_S$ (small), III$_L$ (large), IV, V$_I$ (irregular), V$_N$ (non-structural).

Figure 7. Pitpatterns as visualized on chromoendoscopy

ENDOSCOPIC DIAGNOSIS AND TREATMENT OF EARLY COLORECTAL CANCERS

Endoscopy is the method of choice to detect colorectal neoplasia. While protruding lesions are easily diagnosed, this is more difficult for non-protruding lesions. However, application of modern endoscopic techniques allows detection of non-protruding neoplasia. The most important tools are *chromoendoscopy* (application of 0.2-0.4% indigo karmin dye on the mucosa through the working channel or by a spray catheter) and the use of the 'zoom colonoscope' with magnification power of up to 1:100 [143, 146, 147]. For the diagnosis of *depressed lesions*, slight surface changes (colour changes, bleeding spots, interruption of capillary network pattern, air induced deformation of colonic wall) are important to notice. Then vital stain technique should be applied on such changes. *Flat lesions* are mostly slightly elevated reddish changes. *Laterally spreading tumours* are often difficult to detect without the use of chromoendoscopy.

Kudo et al. [132] described characteristic changes in the surface architecture of the colorectal mucosa (innominate grooves; orifices of colonic crypts) associated with the various types of non-protruding lesions: *pit patterns*. These pit patterns can be visualised clearly by chromoendoscopy. They correlate well with stereo-microscopic examination [148]. Normal pit patterns (type I) can be seen in submucosal lesions (leiomyoma, inflammatory polyps), star-shaped patterns (type II) are associated with hyperplastic polyps. Large tubular (type III_l) and branched (type IV) changes are seen in benign protruded and flat adenomas, while small tubular (type III_s) and irregular (type V_i) or non-structured pit patterns (type V_n) are characteristic for malign depressed lesions. Up to 91% of the invasive lesions have type V_n pit patterns [144].

For the appropriate treatment of colorectal neoplasia, both correct endoscopic diagnosis and histologic-pathological staging are of greatest important. Even if invasion of the submucosa is encountered, some lesions can be treated endoscopically [143, 145, 146, 149]. Small lesions without characteristics like depressed type neoplasia and/or pit patterns suspect for malignancy may be treated by hot biopsy technique.

Protruding lesions are usually removed by endoscopic polypectomy. According to the Haggitt classification (figure 5), up to type III microinvasive cancer can be treated safely with polypectomy alone. Type IV lesions, however, should be treated by surgical resection due to increased risk of lymph node metastases. In sessile rectal adenomas (and even T_1 rectal cancers), transanal endoscopic microsurgery (TEM) is a very suitable method in selected patients [150-153]. Non-protruding lesions can usually be removed by endoscopic mucosal resection (EMR) technique (sm1a + b), while sm1c lesions and beyond should be treated surgically because of increased risk of regional lymph node involvement [149]. The EMR technique is based on elevation of the lesion by injection of 0.9% saline into the submucosa, followed by resection with a snare through the colonoscope, and retrieval of the tissue by an endoscopic forceps. While this technique usually allows removal of lesions up to 20 mm of size, larger polyps can be removed by endoscopic piece-meal resection. Conclusively, improvements in endoscopy techniques and imaging will allow for better detection and minimal-invasive treatment of early colorectal neoplasia and precancers. However, the fundamental for reducing mortality from CRC is prevention of the lesions from developing in the first place.

THE SURROGATE ENDPOINTS BIOMARKER (SEPB)

As a near obligate precursor to cancer, the intraepithelial neoplasia (IEN) is an appropriate target for intervention. Recognized in several epithelial cancers, and occurring in most gastrointestinal epithelial tissues [154-160], IEN shares phenotypic and genotypic similarities with invasive disease and is on the causal pathway leading from normal tissue to cancer. In addition, IEN serves as a significant risk marker for cancer. Subjects with IEN, particularly those with severe IEN, are at significantly higher risk than unaffected individuals for developing invasive cancer in the same tissues. This risk in fact exceeds other measurable factors (*e.g.*, age, race, and family history), with the exception of germ-line mutations that occur in the hereditary genetic syndromes. IEN is also a disease in its own right, in that medical, endoscopic or surgical treatment provides clinical benefit. In standard clinical practice, invasive surgical interventions are used to reduce the burden of IEN, as demonstrated by the use of endoscopic or minimal-invasive techniques, and radical, open surgery methods to treat precursor lesions of the large bowel. This same goal of reducing IEN burden is thus also appropriate for medical (noninvasive) intervention, not only to reduce invasive cancer risk, but also to reduce surgical morbidity.

The colorectal adenoma is an IEN prototype. Whereas IEN is a validated precancer in most epithelial tissues [161-165], colorectal adenomas are one of the best-characterized IENs and a best-case example for using IEN as surrogate end points biomarker (SEPBs) in development of drugs for cancer prevention [166-168]. The adenoma–carcinoma sequence is well characterized. The CRC risk conferred by adenomas is recognized, and screening for and surgical removal of adenomas are already recommended medical practice for prevention of CRC. Further and significantly, strong evidence from epidemiological and clinical studies suggests that drugs that reduce adenoma burden also decrease CRC incidence and mortality. For example, more than 20 studies have demonstrated an association between the frequent use of nonsteroidal anti-inflammatory drugs (NSAIDs), particularly aspirin, and reduced risk of colorectal adenomas, cancers, and cancer-related mortality.

Knowledge of the biology of tumor progression therefore allows us to identify specific tests that are useful for early detection or screening [169]. Molecular probes, for instance, could detect altered DNA shed into the feces [114]. Correlation of the molecular alterations with demographic data, risk factors, environmental exposure, family history, and dietary history may provide important information on the etiology of CRC. Molecular genetic alterations could also contribute toward the assessment of risk. Risk assessment is the search for risk factors that provide the earliest evidence for the risk of cancer in persons not diagnosed with the disease. Biomarkers that are predictive of risk can potentially trigger more aggressive interventions and surveillance. Individuals who test positive for any risk marker become candidates for an intervention or for surveillance. The earliest risk factors are probably the hereditary genetic defects, which is well demonstrated in the case of CRC. However, only a minority of patients shares this genetic predisposition. Thus, a well–defined SEPB, beyond the current use of polyps/adenoma, applicable to the general population at risk for sporadic CRC is highly sought for.

Biomarkers of Risk and Biomarkers for Early Detection

Markers of risk and markers of early detection share the same outcome, namely, the incidence of disease. However, markers of risk and markers for early detection differ in the degree of certainty they convey regarding the existence of cancer. A risk factor confers significantly less than 100% certainty of cancer within a specified time interval, whereas early detection markers confer close to 100% certainty of cancer. Risk markers indicate that cancer is more likely to occur within a specified time in persons with the marker than in the general population. Early detection markers indicate the existence of cancer, or that cancer will occur with nearly a 100% certainty within a specified time interval.

From a screening perspective, all surrogate outcomes in individuals not diagnosed with cancer are risk factors. Colonic polyps, for instance, are a surrogate end point for screening and a risk factor for colon cancer [169, 170]. According to Kelloff and colleagues, at least three elements are necessary to use risk factors as surrogate outcomes in screening:

1 the risk factor and its detection method must be properly defined;
2 the definitive outcome of interest and a description on how to assess it should be indicated; and
3 knowledge of the strength and direction of the relationship between the surrogate outcome and the definitive outcome over a specified time interval should be known.

For a risk factor to be a useful SEPB, it must be strongly connected to the definitive outcome, and the probability and direction of the relationship must be known. Again, several criteria must be met before biomarkers can serve as risk factors or as markers for early detection:

1   the biomarker must be differentially expressed in normal, premalignant or high-risk, and tumor tissue;
2   the marker and its assay must provide acceptable predictive accuracy for risk or for the presence of cancer; and
3   the variance of the detection tests and the intra- and interlaboratory variance must be known.

For biomarkers to serve as SEPBs in prevention interventions, it is necessary to satisfy additional criteria:

1   the marker must be a determinant of outcome;
2   the marker must be modulated by chemopreventive agents; and
3   modulation or elimination of the risk marker must correlate with a decrease in cancer incidence.

Risk markers are usually used as surrogate outcomes to detect the effect of a prevention intervention more rapidly than waiting for the definitive outcome (such as the presence of cancer or not). These criteria can be tested and evaluated in animal models and in human tissue specimens.

There are very few biomarkers for risk of colon cancer, such as colonic adenomas. Biomarkers of risk can be inherited or acquired. With the identification and characterization of inherited defective genes (such as HNPCC and FAP) implicated in the etiology of CRC (figure 2), it has now become possible to identify individuals predisposed to this disease through genetic testing (i.e. microsatellite instability testing, or APC-mutation testing). For this reason, widespread genetic screening will not substantially reduce the incidence of the disease unless additional genes are found. Additional genes may exist because the incidence of colon cancer is 3–4 times higher in families with a history of this disease than in the general population (figure 2). In the search for new ways of characterizing risk in adenomas, our research group has recently identified (by quantitative digitalized image analysis) a *monotonous population of elongated cells* (dubbed MPECs), which discriminate high- from low-risk adenomas at risk for metachronous CRC development better than conventional histology type and grade [171]. The inclusion of immunohistochemistry markers, in particular the anti-apoptosis regulator survivin, the human telomerase reverse transcriptase (hTERT), as well as regulators of the cell cycle ($p16^{INK4A}$ and $p21^{CIP1}$) may further define colorectal adenomas at risk for developing cancer [172]. Clearly, the search for biomarkers will continue to evolve in colorectal carcinogenesis. Likely, increased knowledge of specific cell features, genetic alterations and proteomic characteristics will, in combination, help us identify those patients at particular high risk for cancer development.

Chapter 6

MICROSATELLITE INSTABILITY

Microsatellites are found in great number spread out over the whole DNA sequence and, due to their repetitive manner, are prone to changes during replication. The most common microsatellite in humans is a dinucleotide repeat of cytosine and adenine which occurs in several thousand locations throughout the human germ line [44] (figure 8).

Microsatellite instability is a situation in which a germline microsatellite allele has gained or lost repeated units and has thus undergone a somatic change in length (figure 8). This type of alteration can be detected only if many cells are affected by the same change, and is thus an indicator of the clonal expansion typical of a neoplasm.

Mismatches of nucleotides occur when the DNA-polymerase inserts the wrong bases in the newly synthesized DNA. Normally, when two strands of DNA replicate, nucleotide mismatches occur, but almost all such errors are quickly corrected by a molecular proofreading mechanism (figure 8). The DNA mismatch repair system works as a "spell checker" that identifies and then corrects the mismatched basepairs in the DNA. However, defects in the mismatch repair mechanisms (i.e. mutated genes) lead to MSI. MSI in hereditary and sporadic CRC occurs through two different mechanisms. In HNPCC the cause is a germline mutation in a mismatch-repair enzyme, where alterations of the *MSH2* and *MLH1* mismatch-repair genes account for > 90%. Instability in microsatellite sequences in sporadic CRC MSI is often due to *loss of expression* of the mismatch-repair gene (most commonly *MLH1*) caused by *epigenetic silencing* (see later in this chapter).

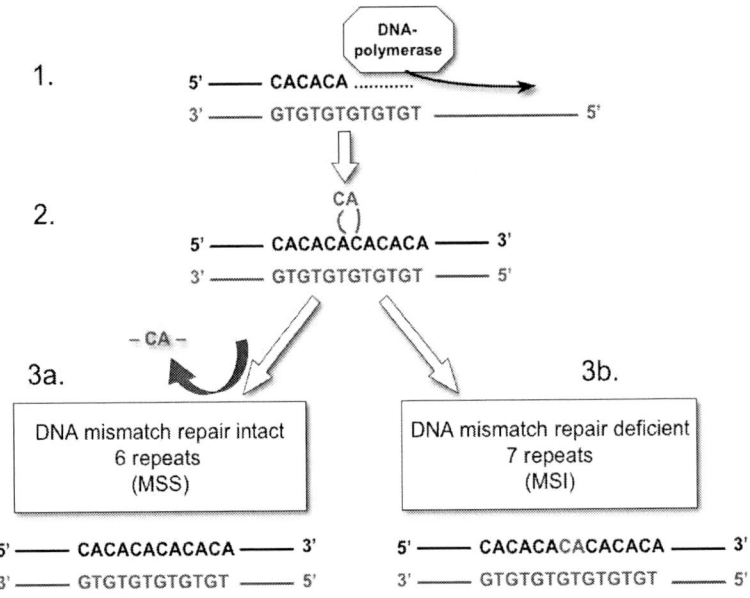

Legend: Mechanism of microsatellite instability (MSI).
(1) Replication of DNA.
(2) A CA repeat erroneously built into the replication strand.
(3a) The error is repaired by mismatch repair enzymes, or
(3b) the error is not repaired causing MSI. Abbreviations denote: MSS, microsatellite stable. A, adenosine; G, guanine; C, cytidine; T, thymidine. The figure is derived from Søreide *et al.* Copyright British Journal of Surgery Society Ltd. Reproduced with permission. Permission is granted by John Wiley & Sons Ltd on behalf of the BJSS Ltd.

Figure 8. DNA-mismatch repair mechanism.

Microsatellite instability was discovered to be a marker in HNPCC a decade ago [44, 50], when searching for LOH in the susceptible region to find a tumour suppressor gene among dinucleotide repeats. Instead, microsatellites that had changed in length were found in all the HNPCCs – not only in the critical genetic region, but virtually everywhere in the genome of the tumour. This phenomenon was termed *"replication error"* and later renamed *"microsatellite instability"*[44, 47, 48, 50]. Widespread MSI in HNPCC is associated with defective DNA-mismatch repair proteins caused by germline mutation of one of the three main genes (*MLH1, MSH2,* and *MSH6*). As a consequence, the lifetime risk for developing CRC is >80% for HNPCC offspring, compared to a lifetime risk for CRC of up to 5-6% in the general population [49, 166]. In addition, the risk is greatly elevated for endometrial cancer (lifetime risk of 50-60%, compared to 2-3% in the general population), moderately increased in ovarian and gastric cancer (12% and 13%, respectively) [49, 173], but equals the normal population for lung, prostate, or breast cancer.

Genetic Differences in CIN and MSI Cancers

Tumours exhibiting CIN and MSI resemble each other in all but a few distinct ways (table 8). Tumours with CIN have mutations in *p53* and *APC*, including gross chromosomal abnormalities. In contrast, tumours with MSI have frameshift mutations in specific target genes, such as *β-catenin* and *TGFβRII* [174], and fewer mutations are found in *k-ras* and *p53* [175]. The genetic variety between MSI and CIN CRCs continues to be explored – considerable "cross talk" between various pathways is encountered (figure 9), although a few differences seem to appear.

The table is derived from Søreide *et al*. Copyright British Journal of Surgery Society Ltd. Reproduced with permission. Permission is granted by John Wiley & Sons Ltd on behalf of the BJSS Ltd.

Defective mismatch repair presumably facilitates malignant transformation by allowing the rapid accumulation of mutations that inactivate genes, which ordinarily have key functions in the cell (table 1, figure 9). The lack of mismatch-repair proteins, fails to correct nucleotide mismatches and thus promotes mutations in other genes. However, genes carrying MSI in their own coding sequences are also involved, such as the *BAX* and *TGFβRII* genes [176]. A frameshift mutation (figure 10) inactivates the *BAX* gene in about 35% of all tumours with MSI. Altered *BAX*-expression is believed to contribute to carcinogenesis by disrupting the apoptosis pathway mediated by *Bcl-2* (figure 9) [177-182]. The *TGFβRII* gene, which encodes *transforming growth factor β (TGF-β) receptor II* [183], undergoes a frameshift in up to 90% of all HNPCC. This mutation leads to a disruption in the function of *TGF-β*, which acts as both a tumour suppressor and promoter in CRC [184-188]. *TGF-β* signalling pathway involves activation of the *Smad* proteins which regulate transcription (figure 9). Other genes with coding microsatellites (i.e. the tumour-suppressor gene $p16^{INK4A}$) are mutated in mismatch-repair–deficient CRC, but their precise roles are not well understood.

Table 8. Genes frequently involved in colorectal cancer

Gene	Chromosome location	Function
APC	5q21-22	Tumour suppressor gene
TGF-βRII	3p22	Cell signalling
MSH2	2p16	DNA mismatch repair
MLH1	3p21	DNA mismatch repair
MSH6	2p16	DNA mismatch repair
K-ras	12p12.1	Oncogene
p53	17p13	Tumour suppressor
Smad2/4	18q21.1	Tumour suppressor
p16^{INK4A}	9p21.3	Cell cycle control
COX2	1q25.2-3	Cell proliferation
DCC	18q21.3	Tumour suppressor gene
Bcl-2	18q21.3	Apoptosis
BAX	19q13.3-4	Apoptosis
MGMT	10q26	DNA repair gene
PTEN	10q23	Tumour suppressor gene

Legend: Abbreviations denote: APC, adenomatous polyposis coli; TGF-βR, transforming growth factor β receptor; MSH, MutB homologue; MLH, MutL homologue; Smad, mothers against decapentaplegic homologue (Drosophila); COX, cyclo-oxygenase; DCC, deleted in colorectal cancer; Bcl, B-cell chronic lymphocytic leukaemia/lymphoma; BAX, Bcl-2-associated X protein; MGMT, O-6-methylguanine DNA methyltransferase; PTEN, phosphatase and tensin homologue.

More recently, the use of array technology has identified a number of genes differentially expressed in the two subtypes of CRC [189-192]. Genomic and proteomic profiles [193] of subtypes of CRC may increase the biological understanding of cancer and hopefully reveal distinct prognostic and predictive markers that can assist clinicians tailor choice and timing of therapy, as well as improve current follow-up regimens [2].

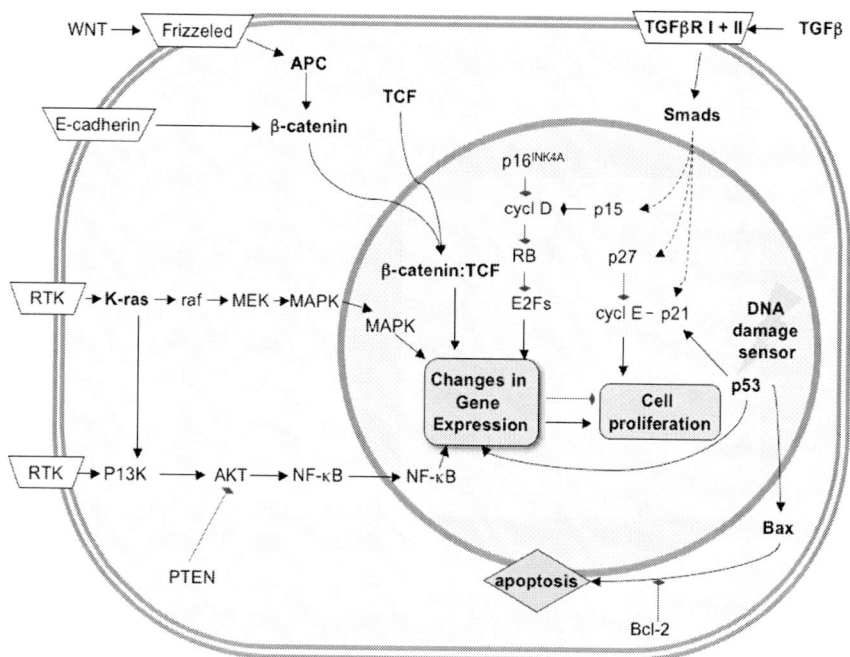

Legend: Simplified overview of general pathways in colorectal cancer. Black arrows suggest a positive interaction; red bars suggest negative control. WNT denotes *Wingless* pathway. AKT, a serine/threonine kinase; APC, adenomatous polyposis coli; BAX, Bcl-2-associated X protein; E2F, E2F transcription factors; MAPK, mitogen-activated protein kinase; MEK, MAPK kinase; NF, nuclear factor; PI3K, phosphatidylinositol 3-kinase; PTEN, phosphatase and tens in homologue; *RB, retinoblastoma* gene; RTK, receptor tyrosine kinase; SMAD, mothers against decapentaplegic homologue (*Drosophila*); TCF, T cell factor; TGF-β(R), transforming growth factor β (receptor).

The figure is derived from Søreide *et al.* Copyright British Journal of Surgery Society Ltd. Reproduced with permission. Permission is granted by John Wiley & Sons Ltd on behalf of the BJSS Ltd.

Figure 9. Colorectal cancer cell-signaling.

Clinicopathological Implications of MSI

Recently, distinct clinical and pathological features (figure 11) of colorectal tumours arising from these two separate mutational pathways have been identified [194-197]. MSI is observed more frequently in women and in CRCs that occur proximal to the splenic flexure. These tumours also exhibit poor differentiation, a mucinous cell type, and frequently peritumoral lymphocytic infiltration ("Crohns-like inflammation") [195, 198, 199]. By which mechanisms this inflammatory response may contribute to the better prognosis remains to be fully explained, but the cytotoxic effects of CD8+ lymphocytes seem to be important [198, 199]. Recent data suggests an interplay with *TGF-β* and peritumoral lymphocytes [184].

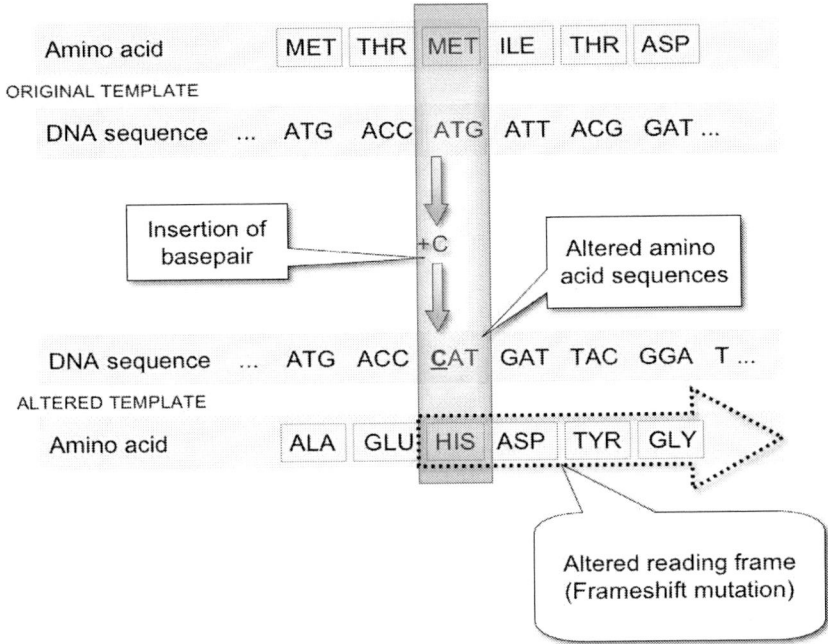

Legend: In a frameshift mutation, the deletion or insertion of a nucleotide shifts the normal sequence of nucleotides in a triplet codon, which may alter the amino acid sequence and thus the protein expressed. In the example, the addition of a base to the DNA sequence shifts the reading frame, such that most amino acids downstream of the alteration are different from those in the original protein. Abbreviations denote:

Deoxyribonucleotides: A, deoxyadenylate; G, deoxyguanylate; C, deoxycytidylate; T, deoxythymidylate. *Amino acids*: Asp, aspartate; Gly, glycine; His, histidine; Ile, isoleucine; Met, methionine; Thr, threonine; Tyr, tyrosine. The figure is derived from Søreide *et al*. Copyright British Journal of Surgery Society Ltd. Reproduced with permission. Permission is granted by John Wiley & Sons Ltd on behalf of the BJSS Ltd.

Figure 10. Frameshift mutations.

Furthermore, MSI tumours are usually diploid unlike the often aneuploid CIN tumours. CRC exhibiting MSI is associated with a larger size (i.e. T_3 tumours) of the primary tumour, but with a more favourable stage distribution (less lymph node involvement and reduced occurrence of metastasis). The pronounced genetic instability of cells with MSI may increase susceptibility to apoptosis because of an accumulation of mutations in genes that are required for cell growth. An increased rate of mutation in other genes might lead to aberrantly expressed proteins in membranes, which may be associated with the antitumour immune response evidenced by the lymphocytic infiltrates that surround tumours with MSI [195, 198, 199]. Clearly, the prognostic benefit of abundant peritumoral infiltration T-cells has been demonstrated in a large cohort of CRCs [68], and correlates with decreased metastatic features, as of yet unexplained reason. As this association continues to be explored, we may experience a change in strategies for staging, prognostication, adjuvant chemotherapy, in addition to new modes of treatment.

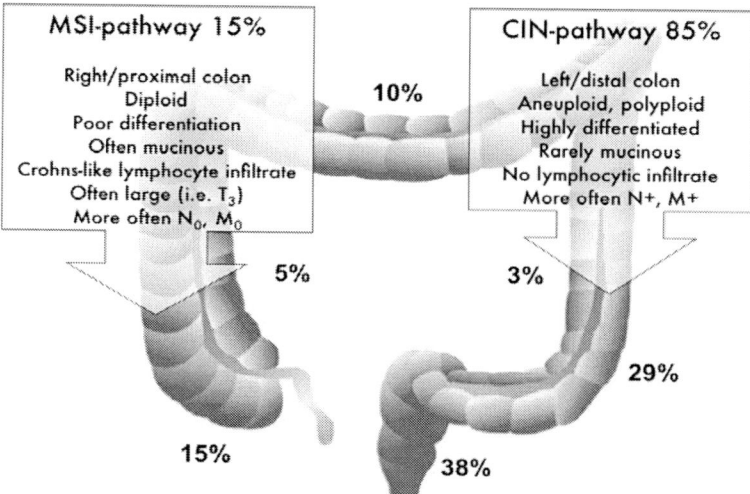

Legend: Pathological distinctions between tumours exhibiting microsatellite instability (MSI) and chromosomal instability (CIN). Percentages indicate the anatomical distribution of colorectal cancers (TNM refers to the tumour node metastasis staging system).

The figure is derived from Søreide *et al*. Copyright British Journal of Surgery Society Ltd. Reproduced with permission. Permission is granted by John Wiley & Sons Ltd on behalf of the BJSS Ltd.

Figure 11. Clinicopathological features of MSI vrs CIN cancers.

MSI cancers have a higher incidence of synchronous and metachronous tumours. Velayos et al [200] explored the MSI patterns in patients with metachronous and synchronous CRC and found that MSI occurred with equal frequency among patients with synchronous and metachronous CRCs. However, the underlying mechanism for MSI was different (loss of *MLH1* expression associated with promoter hypermethylation was more common in MSI-H synchronous CRC). Observed differences in *MLH1* promoter hypermethylation and patient characteristics suggested that most MSI-H synchronous CRCs were sporadic in origin [200].

Most importantly, patients with CRCs that exhibit MSI have longer overall and cancer-specific survival than stage-matched patients with cancers exhibiting CIN [11, 13]. The important contrast in survival between the two types of CRC remains largely unexplained, although links point at inflammatory-related differences. Paradoxically, colorectal cancers with MSI bear many features that are generally associated with poor prognosis, including deep tumor invasion and low histologic differentiation. However, MSI positive tumors are rarely found in hepatic metastasis from CRC [201].

Mutations of the *p53* gene are less frequent in MSI tumors compared with those of the CIN pathway [175]. The same holds true for allelic imbalance at other genetic loci, such as *18q*. Mutations of *p53* are associated with poor prognosis [16], explaining in one way the prognostic advantage of MSI tumors. However, MSI-positive tumors that express *p53* seem to have a more aggressive biology than their *p53*-negative counterparts [194].

Adjuvant chemotherapy with fluorouracil benefit patients with tumors exhibiting CIN, but apparently not those with tumors exhibiting MSI[14]. However, an overall reduced benefit from adjuvant therapy in patients with MSI and CRC could not be demonstrated in a recent systematic review and metaanalysis [13], but the overall survival of MSI colorectal tumors was better. Thus, the mechanism in which MSI tends to render clinically less aggressive cancers remains an interesting but unresolved research target. Real differences in adjuvant chemotherapy response between MSI and CIN tumors remain to be demonstrated. In particular, response-differences should be explored as to the new regimens available in CRC.

Testing for MSI in Colorectal Cancer

The choice of microsatellite markers is important for MSI testing [54, 202-205]. Testing for MSI using the polymerase-chain-reaction (PCR) is straightforward, whereby DNA from the tumour and from normal tissue is tested. Mutations that alter microsatellite length (by deletion or insertion) are visualized as bandshifts on electrophoresis.

The Bethesda Guidelines [53, 206] have proposed a panel of five microsatellite markers for the uniform analysis of MSI in HNPCC. This panel included two mononucleotide (BAT-25 and BAT-26) and three dinucleotide (D5S346, D2S123, and D17S250) repeats. The Bethesda guidelines have since been revised [52], as the use of dinucleotide repeats may cause under– and over–estimation of the instability–status. The revision mainly recommends the use of more mononucleotide markers in unequivocal cases (i.e. in only dinucleotide unstable cases). Screening for HNPCC using the recommended Bethesda MSI markers are now performed in trials for detection of HNPCC [54, 56], however, the current diagnostic yield and implemented costs demand for cautious expectation [55]. Although feasible, the choice to screen all patients with CRC for MSI should await further evidence relating to the clinical importance and therapeutic influence of this information.

Immunohistochemistry (IHC), although proposed to be more cost-effective than PCR, is currently not sensitive and specific enough to be used routinely in detecting MSI in sporadic and hereditary CRC. The reasons for this are several; the heterogeneity within tumors; the weak and focal staining patterns that may be associated with MSI or gene mutation, or both; variability in technical protocols for fixation and staining quality within laboratories; and differences in interpretation of results. The rate of normal IHC results (but with PCR detected mutations) ranges from 2 to 36% in the literature [207-209], and PCR has a higher sensitivity and specificity compared to IHC [210]. One of the major problems with IHC is detection of *MLH1* gene mutations (sensitivity of 44%) – obviously this is of concern as MLH1 is the most frequently altered mismatch repair protein. Consequently, IHC cannot as of yet replace PCR in HNPCC [210].

In a population-based study [207] of sporadic CRC, IHC was evaluated for MSI detection and lacked a positive stain for one or more MMR proteins in about 8% of patients, mostly attributed to *MLH1*. Retesting of discordant cases with both IHC and PCR revealed that IHC failed to detect 17 of 47 MSI cancers [207]. The methods to detect MSI are developing, and correlation with genetic defects explored with cDNA microarray analysis will further improve our understanding in the years to come [191, 203-205, 207, 210-212].

Microsatellite Frequency

For whatever the number of microsatellite markers that are used in a panel, instability in ≥ 40% of markers (i.e. 2 of 5 markers in the Bethesda panel) is defined as *high-frequency* MSI (MSI-H), while instability in 20-40% of markers are defined as *low-frequency* MSI (MSI-L). Tumours with no proven instability (or ≤20%) are termed *microsatellite stable* (MSS) – these tumours comprise those said to follow the CIN-pathway (figure 1). The existence of MSI-L is still controversial and under debate [203, 213-216]. Complexities are related to the wide genomic distribution of dinucleotides, the yet unresolved molecular alterations that have been found in these markers, and the possible influence on carcinogenesis [213, 216-218]. When many dinucleotide markers are used in any chosen panel, a large number of CRC are graded as MSI-L [216]. The select use of mononucleotide markers may avoid this problem [203, 205, 219]. However, proponents of MSI-L tumors have found frequent *k-ras* mutations, as well as more frequently LOH at *5q*, *1p* and *8p* [7], relating them to the CIN-pathway [215] while this has not been confirmed in other studies [216]. Interestingly, some MSI-L tumors are epigenetically silenced in the DNA-repair gene *MGMT* (*O-6-methylguanine DNA methyltransferase*) more frequently than both MSI-H and MSS cancers [220], which may pose a different way to DNA repair errors. MSI-L status has been related to poor prognosis in patients with stage C cancers [15]. Although techniques to more readily detect these subtle differences are developing, such as hypermethylation of *MGMT* [221], the true clinicopathological yield of MSI-L status remains to be established.

Microsatellite Dinucleotides Differences (Type A and B)

The controversy concerning dinucleotide microsatellites does not only pertain to the use of markers. Furthermore, two distinct modes of dinucleotide microsatellite alterations seem to exist in human [217, 218]. Type A alterations are defined as length changes of ≤6 base pairs (bp), while Type B changes are more drastic and involve modifications of ≥8 bp [218]. Defective mismatch repair is necessary and sufficient for Type A changes, and are observed in cell lines and in tumors from mismatch repair gene-knockout mice. In a panel of human colorectal tumors, both Type A and Type B MSI were observed. Both types of MSI were associated with *MSH2* or *MLH1* mismatch repair gene alterations. Intriguingly, *p53* mutations (generally regarded as uncommon in MSI tumors) were frequently associated with Type A instability [217], whereas none were found in tumors with Type B instability, reflecting the prevailing viewpoint. The observation that type A MSI is associated with *p53* mutation in human CRC may be compatible with reports that have shown a connection between *p53* mutation and the MSI-L phenotype, since in CRC Type A MSI tends to be observed in a limited number of markers and, consequently, categorized as MSI-L. MSI observed in various malignancies, including those associated with HNPCC, is predominantly Type B. This may indicate that Type B instability is not a simple reflection of a repair defect. Rather, there may be at least two qualitatively distinct modes of dinucleotide MSI in human CRC, and different molecular mechanisms may underlie these modes of MSI. The relationship between MSI and defective mismatch repair may thus be more complex than hitherto suspected.

Chapter 7

EPIGENETIC SILENCING

Classically, cancer has been viewed as a set of diseases that are driven by progressive, step–by–step, multiple genetic abnormalities that include mutations in tumor-suppressor genes and oncogenes, and chromosomal abnormalities. However, it is apparent that cancer is also a disease that is driven by 'epigenetic changes' — patterns of altered gene expression that are mediated by mechanisms that do not affect the primary DNA sequence [222-225]. These epigenetic alterations occur within a larger context of extensive alterations to chromatin in neoplastic cells in comparison with the normal cells from which they are derived. These involve both losses and gains of DNA methylation as well as altered patterns of histone modifications. Although the molecular determinants that underlie these types of chromatin change in neoplastic cells are only beginning to be elucidated, the best understood component is the transcriptional repression of a growing list of tumor–suppressor and candidate tumor–suppressor genes. This suppression is associated with abnormal methylation of DNA at certain cytosine residues of the cytosine and guanine rich regions called *CpG islands* that often lie in the promoter regions of these genes. *CpG islands* are regions of DNA that are often located proximally to the transcription start site of genes that contain a high frequency of CG dinucleotides. In most mammalian genes, these regions are normally maintained free of DNA methylation, or may an epigenetic mechanism that represses gene transcription in normal cellular processes. In cancer cells, CpG islands in various tumor–suppressor genes are frequently densely methylated, which results in repression of transcription.

By this mechanism of 'silencing', the expression of these tumor–suppressor genes in the cancer cell can be reduced or eliminated as an alternative mechanism to genetic mutation. The increasing recognition of the importance of epigenetic changes in cancer pathogenesis has led to a shift in the approaches that are used to discover genes that are affected by this process [226, 227]. The field has moved from studying the effects of silencing on classic tumor–suppressor genes to searching for candidate tumor–suppressor genes, on the basis of the hypermethylation of promoter regions. In fact, random searches of the cancer-cell genome are now being carried out to detect changes in methylation and chromatin status, either overall or in specific regions of the genome. The identification of genes that are specifically hypermethylated (which results in gene silencing) or hypomethylated (which results in increased transcription) might lead to the discovery of new factors that are important for neoplasia initiation and progression. Of particular importance is the identification of genes, the silencing of which confers a survival benefit to the cells, contributing to a neoplastic phenotype and facilitating neoplasia progression by allowing the accumulation of additional genetic and/or epigenetic hits. Genome methylation patterns are also being developed as biomarkers for tumor type, as markers for risk assessment, early detection and monitoring of prognosis, and as indicators of susceptibility or response to therapy [228-230].

Recently, epigenetic alterations have been shown to occur in colon polyps and colon cancers. The aberrant methylation of genes appears to co-operate with the genetic alterations to drive the initiation and progression of colon polyps to colon cancer. These hypermethylated genes are not only probable pathogenic events affecting colorectal cancer formation, but also neoplasm-specific molecular events that may be useful as molecular markers for colon tumors. Furthermore, aberrant DNA methylation of tumor–suppressor genes may occur secondary to a genetic predisposition or to a field–cancerization effect in the colon and may be useful as molecular markers for the risk of developing CRC.

As previously stated in this chapter, deficient DNA mismatch repair (leading to microsatellite instability) occurs in approximately 15% of all sporadic CRC. In contrast to HNPCC cases, the cause in sporadic CRC is often bi–allelic or hemi–allelic [231] methylation of the CpG-rich promoter sequences of *MLH1* [231-234]. Simply stated, the 'epigenetic change' affect gene function (without genetic changes) by aberrant methylation of DNA that prevents the gene (-region) from being transcribed, thus 'silences' the gene, and cause deficiency in protein expression. Epigenetic silencing is now recognized as a 'third pathway' in Knudson's model of tumour-suppressor gene inactivation in cancer [192, 235]. For selected genes, epigenetic changes are tightly related to neoplastic transformation in CRC. As an example, loss of the tumour suppressor gene *PTEN* located at *10q23* occurs through promotor hypermethylation in CRC with MSI-H [190]. In the large bowel, aberrant DNA methylation arises very early, initially in normal mucosa, and may be part of the age-related field defect observed in sporadic CRC. Aberrant methylation also contributes to later stages of CRC formation and progression through a hypermethylator phenotype termed *CpG Island Methylator Phenotype* (CIMP). CIMP appears to be a defining event in up to half of all sporadic CRCs [236] (figure 1). CIMP-positive CRCs are distinctly characterized by pathological, clinical and molecular genetic features [236-239].

MSI in sporadic CRC usually arises because of epigenetic silencing of the DNA mismatch repair gene *MLH1* [240], and is thus associated with methylation, but the overlap of "mutator" and "methylator" phenotypes is not exact [28, 41, 43]. In particular, some cancers with extensive DNA methylation do not show the mutator phenotype. Although DNA methylation is associated with a worse outcome in CRC, this adverse prognostic influence is lost in methylated tumours with MSI [241]. Collectively these factors add a layer of complexity to the molecular classification of CRC.

The Serrated Adenoma

Serrated adenomas (SA) of the colorectum show features intermediate between hyperplastic polyps (HP) and adenomas. HP and SA are related lesions and there is now strong evidence for a *'serrated-polyp pathway'* to colorectal cancer (CRC) that is largely independent of the classic adenoma-to-carcinoma sequence [59, 242-252]. A recently recognized lesion in this pathway is a HP variant characterized by relatively large size, atypical histology and proximal location in the colorectum [245, 252, 253]. This HP variant has been given a variety of names in the literature, including 'sessile SA' and 'type I SA'. SAs are characterized by a heterogeneous group of changes at the molecular level, but a high proportion have *B-raf* mutations and DNA methylation. They may develop in HP or sessile serrated polyps, or may arise *de novo*. In the serrated polyp pathway, the advent of genetic instability is likely to be an important rate–limiting step that drives rapid neoplastic evolution. Methylation and inactivation of the DNA repair genes *MLH1* and *MGMT* have been proposed as critical steps leading to genetic instability [242, 243] with about one third of all SA being microsatellite instable tumors [250]. It is possible that many, if not all, CRCs with the CIMP phenotype evolve through the serrated-polyp pathway that would, therefore, explain approximately 20% of all CRCs. The current lack of guidelines for managing serrated polyps may explain the static incidence of proximal CRC, despite the falling incidence rates for left-sided CRC during the last decades.

The entity of serrated adenoma of the colorectum was first proposed in 1990 [254] and is thus a relatively new precursor aspect within colorectal neoplasia. The serrated adenoma was characterized as an epithelial neoplasia combining the architectural features of a hyperplastic polyp with the cytological features of an adenoma [254, 255]. Over the past few years, various clinicopathological studies on serrated adenoma have been reported, but its histogenesis remains unclear [136, 243, 248, 256-258]. The inclusion of a "serrated neoplasia pathway" leading to malignancy, which is different from the so-called adenoma-carcinoma sequence, has been adopted in the colorectal carcinogenetic stepwise genetic model. As research evolve, new findings and pathogenetic steps will bring us further to novel techniques of prevention diagnosis and therapy.

Chapter 8

CYCLOOXYGENASE-2 AND COLORECTAL NEOPLASIA

Over the last 20 years, there has been paid increasing attention to the role of prostaglandins in colorectal cancer. The selective COX-2 inhibitors (coxibs) have contributed considerably to the detailed understanding of the mechanisms of PG in the cellular processes in CRC. The role of PGs in evolution of CRC has convincingly been established through multidisciplinary study model, including epidemiological studies [259], randomized trials [260-263] pharmacological intervention in animal models [264, 265] and transgenic mice [266, 267], and in cell-lines [268, 269]. The message carried from these studies suggests that prostaglandins (induced by COX) play a crucial role in development of neoplasmic changes in the colonic epithelium [270, 271], which is reversed by NSAIDs or coxibs [271-273].

COX-2 IN COLORECTAL CARCINOGENESIS

In the adenoma–carcinoma sequential model (figure 1), mutation of the APC gene represents one of the first genetic events. Consequently, the interplay between *APC* mutations and COX-2 activation/inhibition has been examined [274-278]. *COX-2* expression temporally follows the APC gene mutation, indicating that involvement of COX-2 pathways is important in the carcinogenesis [279]. Exact how the mutant *APC* activates the *COX-2* gene remains to be elucidated, but recent experiments in the Zebra fish indicate that *APC* activates *COX-2* expression via the transcription factor C/EBP-β and retinoic acid [274].

Regulation of *COX-2* expression is complex and includes inflammatory stimuli, cytokines, hormones and tumor promoters [280]. Several of these factors merge on pathways that have response elements in the promoter region of the *COX-2* gene, such as cAMP, NF-kB, NF-IL6, and E-box [281]. Moreover, epigenetic modulation of *COX-2* is common, and hypomethylation may be found in >70% of CRCs [282].

Posttranslational regulation of COX-2 protein production is essential. The transcribed m-RNA is of no use if it is not translated into the protein. Increased COX-2 messenger RNA (mRNA) stability by reduction of its decay by a RNA binding protein seems to be of importance [283, 284]. Furthermore, increased translation of the COX-2 mRNA may be enhanced through the K-ras/PKB1 pathway [285] and decreased by the translation silencer TIA-1 [286]. The regulation of the amount of active COX-2 protein is obviously complex and dependent on interplay of a vast number of factors on different levels.

PROSTAGLANDINS AND PROSTAGLANDIN RECEPTORS

Prostaglandins are locally produced hormones with a diversity in structure and function, and exerts their effects locally in a autocrine and paracrine manner[287]. Arachidonic acid is the precursor and cyclooygenase (COX) /PGH synthase is the rate limiting step in the synthesis [288]. The two isoforms of this enzyme, denoted COX-1 and COX-2, share functions where COX-1 is the housekeeping cytoprotective enzyme while COX-2 is inducible to inflammation and neoplasm [289, 290]3[289, 291]. The intermediate product, PGH_2, is rapidly converted by specific enzymes to prostaglandins and tromboxanes (figure 12).

Cox-2 is not expressed in normal colonic epithelium, but is upregulated in 40-50 % of adenomatous polyps, and 80-90 % in CRC [271, 287, 292, 293]. Also, it is upregulated due to inflammatory stimuli in ulcerative colitis patients [294], who have a selective 5-7 fold increased risk of CRC [76]. In the colonic epithelium, PGE_2 is the main PG-product of COX-2 upregulation [295, 296]. PGE_2 produced in the epithelial cell is transported through special PG-transporters [297] out to the exterior of the cell where it creates the autocrine and paracrine effects (figure 12). Also, an isomer of secretory PLA_2 ($sPLA_2$-X) secreted into the juxta cellular microenvironment may liberate free arachidonic acid from the outer part of the cell membrane[298]. Hence, the COX-2 expression in the tumor stroma [299] may produce prostaglandins (included PGE_2) and increase the micro environmental PGE_2 amount.

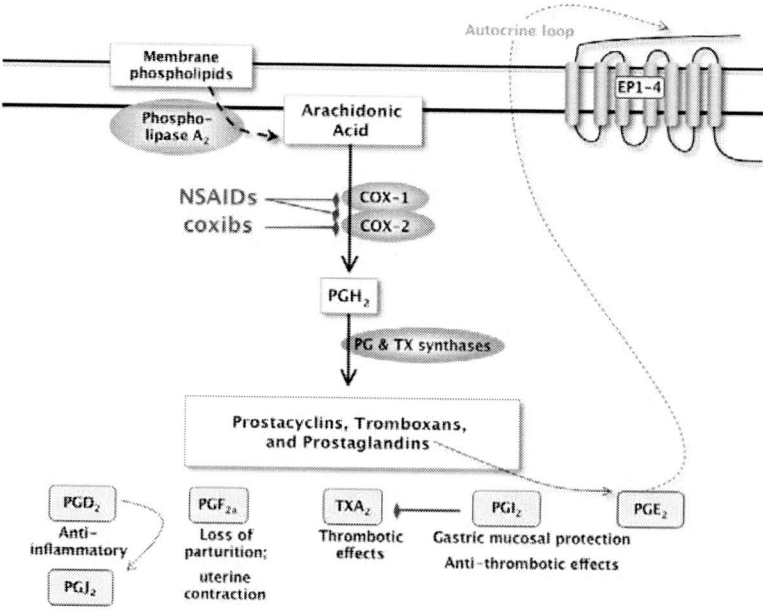

Legend: COX, cyclooxygenase; NSAIDs, non-steroidal anti-inflammatory drugs; PG, prostaglandin; TX, tromboxans

Figure 12. Eicosanoid synthesis.

The PGE_2 exerts its effect through four different 7-trans-membrane G-coupled receptors, EP_1, EP_2, EP_3 and EP_4 that activate important downstream second messenger systems [300] (figure 12 and figure 13). The effect of the PGE_2 on the colon epithelial cells will depend on the relative distribution and grade of expression of these receptors. Due to the cross talk between pathways, the transcription of the *COX-2* gene is further increased, and a positive augmentation loop is established. This is in line with increasing COX 2 expression from adenoma level to carcinoma level [287].

It is important to distinguish the effects of PGE_2 downstream signal pathways and the effect of NSAIDs and COX-2 inhibitors (coxibs), since the latter inhibit a broader specter of PGs, not only PGE_2. Prostaglandines, particularly the PGE_2, contribute to several of the "hallmark" features in carcinogenesis [22] and increased knowledge in this field may give way for new, targeted areas of therapy beyond the current effects of NSAIDs or coxibs.

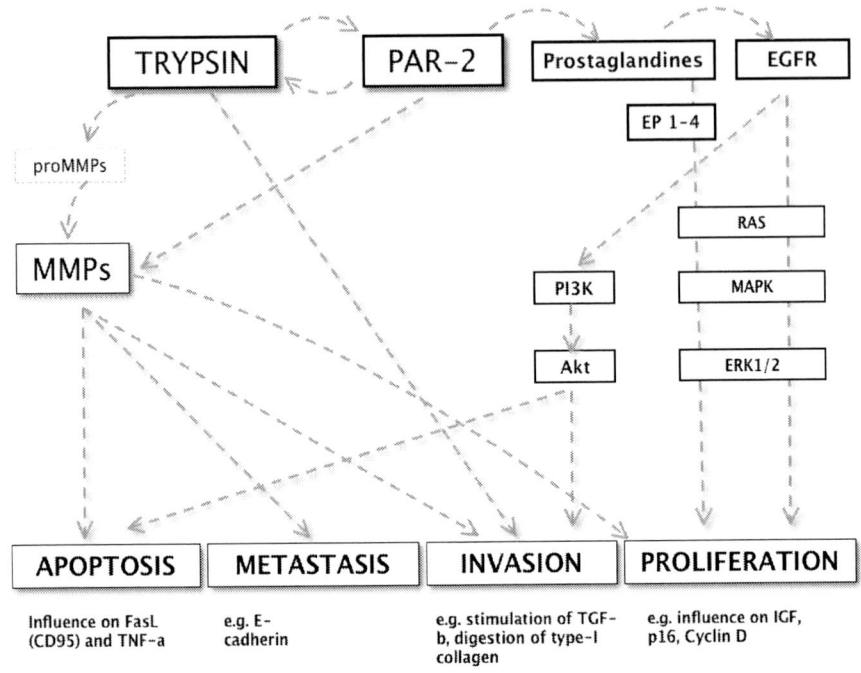

Figure 13. Interplay between various protease-systems and cancerogenesis.

Self-Sufficiency of Growth Signals

Mutation in the APC gene is one of the earliest event in both familiar adenomatous polyposis syndrome and sporadic CRC [61]. The molecular effect of this mutation is decreased phosphorylation and hence decreased degradation of β-catenin, which increases the β-catenin level and enhance the cell proliferation through the Wnt-Frizzled pathways [301]. Castellone and colleagues [302] have shown that PGE_2 stimulates colon cancer cell growth through its heterotrimeric G protein-coupled receptor, EP2, by a signaling route that involves the activation of phosphoinositide 3-kinase (PI3K) and the protein kinase Akt by free G protein betagamma subunits and the direct association of the G protein alphas subunit with the *regulator of G protein signaling* (RGS) domain of axin. This leads to the inactivation and release of *glycogen synthase kinase 3β* (GSK-3β) from its complex with axin, thereby relieving the inhibitory phosphorylation of β-catenin and activating its signaling pathway. This in turn, leads to increased stable dephosphorylated β-catenin[302, 303] and increased levels of *c-myc* and cyclin D1[304, 305].

Further, PGE2 acts via EP2 and EP4 receptors, and on the *epidermal growth factor receptor* (EGFR) and Akt pathways[306, 307]. Activation Ras mediate signaling trough the MAPK- patway [308]. Also, cAMP is upregulated through EP2 /EP4 and increase the activation of ligands related to EGFR [309]

PI3K is activated by EP2/EP4 and activates the Akt- pathway downstream. In addition, there is a transactivating augmentation of each pathway. Both the cAMP/PKA and the Akt-pathway increase phosphorylation of GSK-3β and its release from axin, hence enhance the β-catenin pathway. In turn, both MAPK and β-cathenin:TCF complex increase the COX-2 transcription, contributing to the self sufficiency of proliferation and growth signals [307, 310].

Evation of Apoptosis

An important contribution to cell survival due to PGE_2 is the inhibition of mitochondrial associated apoptosis [299, 311, 312]. This means increase of bcl-2 followed by reduced cytochrome-c release and attenuated caspase 9 and 3 [287]. This mechanism is both detected in human and Rat intestinal epithelial cells [313, 314]. In cholangiocarcinoma, it is shown that COX-2 inhibitors inhibits FAS-mediated apoptosis, explained by PGE_2 up regulation of Mcl-1, a protein in the bcl-2 family [315]. The crosstalk between the Akt-pathway in interacting with Bcl-2[316], is of importance for apoptotic control.

Moreover, inhibition of COX-2 enhances proteosomal degradation of Survivin. This indicates that PG increase survival and inhibition of apoptosis [317]. In addition, there is a complex relationship between p53, NF-kB and COX-2 expression [318], where p53 seems to increase COX-2 expression via NF-kB. Consequently, when a epithelial cell has undergone DNA damage, p53 is activated in order to slow down cell cycle progression and thus allow for DNA repair mechanisms to interfere. Parallel to this, the COX-2 and PGE_2 pathways are activated to keep the cell alive and not let it enter apoptosis [72].

Sustained Angiogenesis

The angiogenetic switch takes place when the balance between angiogenetic inhibitors and pro-angiogenetic factors (such as IL–8, TNF–α, and *vascular endothelial growth factor*, VEGF) [319] turn in favor of neo-angiogenesis. IL–1β from macrophages in the invasive front promotes transcription of several proangiogenic factors, including COX-2. PGE_2 contributes to the angiogenesis by increasing the transcription of HIF-1α, which in turn increases production of VEGF [320], and by activating the ERK-Jnk pathway [287].

The prostaglandin-role in CRC continues to evolve. As delineated in the further sections, prostaglandin co-acts with several other protease systems. Consequently, some of these events will be illuminated further.

Chapter 9

TRYPSIN IN COLORECTAL CANCER

Trypsin is one of the best-characterized serine proteinases. Proteases play essential roles in many physiological processes (i.e. food digestion, blood coagulation, fibrinolysis, and control of blood pressure) but also in a wide range of important pathological processes (i.e. atherosclerosis, inflammation, and cancer) [321, 322].

Previously trypsin was known as a digestive enzyme primarily produced by pancreatic acinar cells. However, the presence of trypsin in pancreatectomized patients led to investigation of production at other sites in the human body [323]. Currently, trypsin expression in epithelial cells of skin, esophagus, stomach, small intestine, colon, lung, kidney, liver, bile ducts, as well as leukocytes, and splenic and neuronal cells has been documented [324]. Four different trypsinogen isoforms have been characterized in humans; trypsinogen-1, trypsinogen-2, trypsinogen-3 (found in various epithelial tissues), and trypsinogen-4 (found in the brain) [325-327]. The different trypsinogens show great homology (>90%) at both nucleotide and protein level.

Trypsin has a very proteolytic activity selectively against the peptide bonds in protein molecules that have carboxyl groups donated by the amino acids *arginine* and *lysine*. For physiological protection against premature activity, as known from pancreatic physiology, trypsin is secreted as an inactive zymogen (trypsinogen) in the pancreatic juice, and is activated into trypsin through an enteropeptidase in the alkaline milieu of the duodenal lumen. Secondly, trypsinogen requires activation into active trypsin by a enteropeptidase found in duodenal enterocytes [328]. Of interest, adenocarcinoma cells of the duodenum [328], as well as other tissues expressing trypsin, have a trypsin-activating enteropeptidase [329]. Lastly, the anti-protease mediator *pancreatic secretory trypsin inhibitor* (PSTI) protects from premature activity. An imbalance in this protease/anti-protease system plays a pathophysiological role in the development of pancreatitis [330, 331], and seems to pose an increased risk for developing pancreatic adenocarcinoma [332]. PSTI is excreted by mucosa of the normal gastrointestinal tract where it serves to protect the cells from proteolytic breakdown. The same peptide is secreted by tumor cells, and is often referred to as "tumor-associated trypsin inhibitor" (TATI), identical to the PSTI [333].

GENERAL ASPECTS OF TRYPSIN IN CANCER

Trypsin expression is increased in human cancer cells of the ovary [334, 335], prostate [336], lung [337], stomach [338], colon [339, 340], and others [339, 341]. Trypsin in cancer is often referred to as "tumour-associated trypsin" (TAT), and generally represents trypsin-1 and trypsin-2 [335, 336, 342-345].

The contributing role of the tumor environment and its constituents (i.e. stroma cells, signal molecules, matrix enzymes) in the invasive and metastatic process is emerging (figure 3) [346-349]. Trypsin, as a matrix serine proteinase, has an evolving role in the understanding of this process, as evident by the poor prognosis in patients with overexpression of trypsin [335, 336, 340, 350]. Current evidence suggest the adverse effect to be mediated through an interplay with other protease-systems (figure 3), such as the matrix metalloproteinases (MMPs) [329, 333, 341, 345, 351-354] and the recently explored proteinase-activated receptor 2 (PAR-2) [355-357]. The role of these proteinase-cascade systems and their mutual contribution to cancer development remains elusive, but knowledge is evolving.

The current mechanisms by which trypsin induces invasion and metastasis seems to be manifold (figure 13). First, as a proteolytic enzyme, trypsin may directly degrade extracellular proteins by itself, i.e. by attacking type 1 collagen of the basal membrane [345]. Secondly, its effect is likely indirectly mediated through the activation and effect of other latent proteolytic cascades, the most important ones being the MMPs. Lastly, recent evidence points at the activation of signal molecules, such as proteinase-activated receptor 2 (PAR-2).

The Role of Trypsin in Colorectal Cancer

Trypsin overexpression correlates with poor prognosis in patients with CRC, a fact that has been established through several lines of evidence. For one, Yamamoto and colleagues [340] found trypsin immunoreactivity to be more intense at the invasive front than in the superficial part of the tumor. Trypsin positivity (arbitrarily defined as >30% positive cells at the invasive front of CRCs) significantly correlated with depth of invasion, lymphatic and venous invasion, lymph node and distant metastasis, advanced pathological tumour-node-metastasis (TNM) stage, as well as recurrence. Trypsin activates matrilysin (MMP-7), which plays an important role in CRC progression, and may explain the adverse effect of trypsin on CRC prognosis. Patients with positive stains for both trypsin and matrilysin fared the worst [340].

Furthermore, a Northern blot analysis[358] of RNA isolated from a series of 28 malignant colon tumors and corresponding normal mucosa showed that trypsinogen transcripts were up-regulated 2- to 33-fold in about one third of CRC. Trypsinogen mRNA was expressed in 6 colorectal cancer cell lines, with highest levels detected in the metastatic tumor cell lines [358]. Immunostaining for trypsinogen protein expression showed intense immunoreactivity in the supranuclear cytoplasm of colon tumors in 16% of tissue specimens. To evaluate the relative contributions of 2 isoforms of trypsinogen-1 and -2 to total trypsinogen mRNA expression, a semi-quantitative multiplex reverse-transcriptase-polymerase-chain reaction (RT-PCR) assay was developed [358]. Trypsinogen-2 mRNA was detected in all 6 colorectal tumor cell lines, whereas trypsinogen-1 mRNA was expressed only in the metastatic tumor lines, showing that the high levels of trypsinogen expression in the metastatic tumor lines are likely due to up-regulation of trypsinogen-1. Williams et al [358] suggest that trypsinogen-2 is the dominant trypsinogen in colon tissue and up-regulation of trypsinogen-1 expression in colon tumors may be associated with a metastatic phenotype.

Similar results have been achieved by Solakidi et al [359] examining qualitatively and semi-quantitatively the immunohistochemical expression of trypsin and TATI on paraffin-embedded serial tissue sections from 91 CRCs, with RT-PCR also performed on fresh tissues in 55 of the cases. Normal and non-malignant tissues adjacent to the tumors were also evaluated. Cytoplasmic expression of trypsin (defined as > 25% of the cancer cells positive) was found in 67 (74%) adenocarcinomas, whereas TATI was expressed in the cytoplasm of 59 (65%). Trypsin and TATI correlated significantly in immunohistochemical expression ($p<0.01$). RT-PCR showed co-expression of trypsin and TATI mRNA in all CRC. Distinct patterns of trypsin and TATI immunohistochemical expression were observed in adjacent, non-malignant tissues, where both trypsin and TATI mRNA were also detected. Normal tissues were negative by immunohistochemistry.

In addition to conclusions drawn from other studies [340, 358], Solakidi demonstrated the co-expression of trypsin and TATI in colorectal tumors both at the mRNA and protein level [359]. Controversially, trypsin in oesophageal and gastric cancers may have a tumor-suppressive effect [360], but this is in stark contrast to studies reported for several other cancer types, including CRC [335, 336, 340, 345, 359, 361, 362].

Trypsin as a Target for Therapy

Cancer cells show an analogy to the natural protective mechanisms of trypsin by expressing an trypsin inhibitor (tumor-associated trypsin inhibitor; TATI) at increased levels in CRCs compared to adjacent normal mucosa [339, 341, 359, 363-366]. This suggests an innate protective mechanism occurring even in tumours.[365] Although TATI is highly coexpressed in CRC, experimental inhibition of trypsin with TATI is only partial successful,[345] and nor does TATI serve as a useful tumor marker compared to carcino-embryonic antigen (CEA).[367] Inhibition of trypsin mediated invasion has been performed by using derivatives of tetracyclines [344]. However, trypsin interacts with other cascades, making single-targeted inhibition difficult and likely ineffective. At present, inhibition of trypsin to reduce the cancer progression seems unsuccessful, but success may derive from more specific inhibitors and increased knowledge of the cascades coactivated in CRC.

Chapter 10

OTHER PROTEINASE-SYSTEMS

There are two major proteinase cascades which are directly activated by trypsin, namely the matrix metalloproteinases (MMPs) and the proteinase-activated receptor 2 (PAR2). The contribution of these cascades to proliferation, invasion, and metastasis has just recently been recognized (figure 13). The following paragraphs will appreciate trypsin with this connection in further detail.

TRYPSIN ACTIVATES MATRIX METALLOPROTEINASES (MMP)

MMPs and serine proteinases are the two major groups of proteinases. MMPs are extensively studied in cancer [321, 322, 350, 368-370]. Trypsin activates a number of pro-collagenases, including MMP-1, MMP-8, and MMP-13,[345] MMP-7,[340] MMP-2 and MMP-9 [342]. Trypsin activated MMP-9 stimulates the invasiveness in tongue cancers.[354] Trypsin may initiate proteolytic cascades further enhanced by MMPs. Several MMPs have proved to induce progression, invasion and induction of metastasis in CRC [338, 347, 352, 371-383].

The role of MMPs in CRC has recently been reviewed elsewhere [350, 368, 369]. Trypsin acts in concert with MMPs. Overexpression of several MMPs (MMP-1, -2, -3, -7, -8, -9, -10, -12, -13, -14) has been found in CRC, of which MMP-2, MMP-7, and MMP-9 are co-expressed together with trypsin and seem to be of special importance concerning proliferation, progression, and invasion [340, 347, 351, 368, 373, 384, 385]. MMPs may play a role in both conversion from adenoma to carcinoma, and in the initiation of invasion and metastasis.[350, 368, 371] The degree of over-expression of some MMPs has been noted to correlate with stage of disease and prognosis.[340, 351, 371, 386, 387] Whether MMPs are produced by the stromal cells surrounding a tumor, or by the cancer cells themselves continues to be debated (figure 3). Evidence suggests, however, that co-segregation of trypsin and MMPs within the tumor environment is important for the activation of MMPs, and thus explain the deleterious role of trypsin on prognosis in CRC [340, 351, 352, 354, 372].

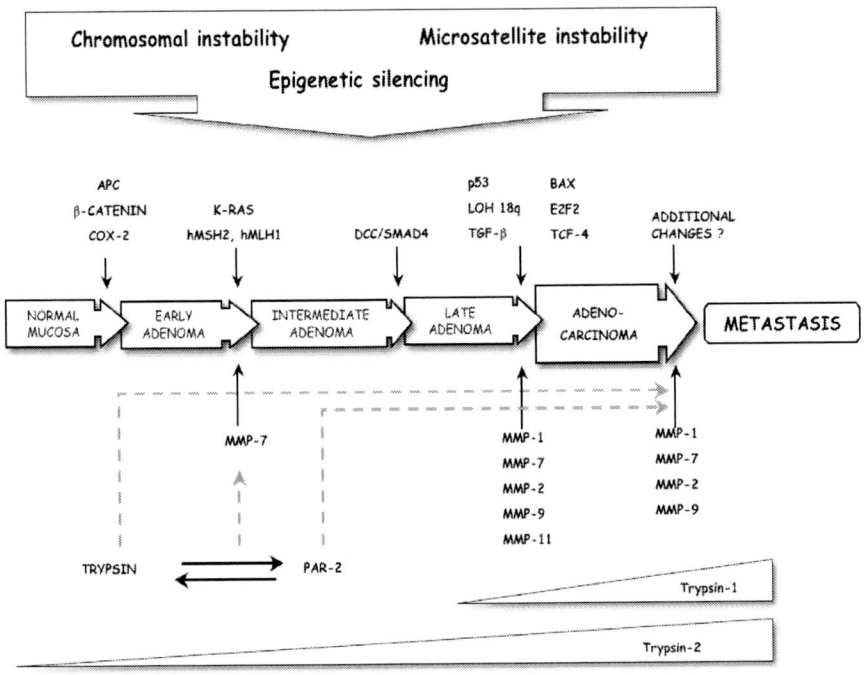

Legend: Developed from Søreide et al [20].

Figure 14. Trypsin, MMPs and PAR-2 in the colorectal progression model.

The role of MMPs has evolved through the last three decades; they seem to play a role in the transition from adenoma to carcinoma, are influenced by certain mutational patterns (such as APC mutation), and are less likely found in CRCs with microsatellite instability and a favorable prognosis [368, 388, 389]. Successful experimental inhibition of MMPs has led to initiation of several human trials. However, the human trials have failed to reproduce the experimental inhibitory effects on cancer growth [370]. Most trials have been based on patients with advanced pancreatic or gastric cancer; subjects probably beyond therapeutic effect [370]. Thus, new surrogate endpoints have been called for, such as the ability to prevent new development of adenomas; effect on regression of adenomas; or inhibition of the progression of adenomas to carcinomas [369].

The evidence of trypsin activation of pro-MMPs suggests that trypsin may play a role, however indirectly, in colorectal cancer progression even in the early development from adenoma to carcinoma (figure 14). Consequently, further elaboration of the biological role trypsin and MMPs in early stage CRC is warranted.

TRYPSIN AND PROTEINASE ACTIVATED RECEPTORS (PARs)

Seven transmembrane G-protein-coupled receptors comprise the biggest group of receptors in mammalian systems, and a large number of cognate receptors and associated ligands have been identified. A recently described novel subset of this group, the proteinase-activated receptors (PARs), has unique mechanism of activation [390, 391]. Rather than being activated by simple ligand occupancy, they are activated enzymatically through proteolysis of the receptor. This proteolytic cleavage is specifically mediated by the serine proteases, such as thrombin (for PAR-1) and trypsin (for PAR-2) [392, 393].

Classically, serine proteases have been shown to play important roles in diverse biological functions, particularly in relation to clot formation and wound healing. However, proteolytic cleavage of PARs as a mode of receptor activation now represents an increasingly important feature of this family of enzymes [390].

PAR-2 is the second of the four "PAR" members characterized by proteolytic cleavage of an amino terminus, thus exposing a tethered peptide ligand that autoactivates the receptor [394]. Although traditionally thought of as degrading enzymes, these proteinases function as signal molecules at the cell surface [391]. PAR-2 is expressed in numerous cell types within the gastrointestinal tract, suggesting both multiple functions and numerous modes of receptor activation. PAR-2 activation induce an effect on epithelial ion-transport [395, 396]. PAR-2 is strongly expressed in enterocytes in both basolateral and apical membranes [394].

PAR-2 and PAR-1 have several common functions. Both receptors contribute to growth regulation and mitogenesis. Both receptors also induce endothelium-dependent relaxation of coronary artery and aortic smooth muscle, resulting in hypotension. In the gastrointestinal tract, PAR-2 may influence motility, since its activation results in contraction of gastric muscle.

Very high expression of PAR-2 has been found in certain tumour cell lines derived from the lung, colon, and pancreas. Pancreas cancer cell lines containing PAR-2 proliferate upon exposure to trypsin, whereas cancer cell lines not containing PAR-2 fails to proliferate upon trypsin expression [397]. This suggests that the presence of PAR-2 is needed for trypsin to induce proliferation in cancer cells.

TRYPSIN ACTIVATION OF PAR-2 IN AN AUTOCRINE LOOP

Proteinase-activated receptor 2 (PAR-2) is activated by trypsin [362, 396, 398]. In fact, trypsin functions as the strongest activator of PAR-2 [398]. Conversely, PAR-2 has also been reported to activate trypsin, which suggest an autocrine activating loop (figure 13) between the two [362]. Trypsin-induced PAR-2 activation has a proliferative effect on CRC cells,[355] and thus a mitogenic role for PAR-2 mediated by trypsin has been proposed in CRC growth (figures 13 and 14) [399]. Furthermore, PARs 1 and 2 contribute to tumour cell motility and metastasis [400]. Factors contributing to the biological cascade under which PAR-2 takes action to induce cell growth has recently been proposed [357]. PAR-2 up-regulates interleukin-8 and contribute to cancer cell migration [401].

TRYPSIN INDUCES PROLIFERATION BY PAR-2

Evidence suggest trypsin-induced proliferation in CRC by activation of PAR-2 by the following mechanisms (figures 13 and 14): (a) a MMP-dependent release of transforming growth factor (TGF)-α, as demonstrated with TGF-α-blocking antibodies and measurement of TGF-α in culture medium; (b) TGF-α-mediated activation of epidermal growth factor receptor (EGFR) and subsequent EGFR phosphorylation; and (c) activation of ERK1/2 and subsequent cell proliferation [357]. The link between these events is demonstrated by the fact that stimulation of cell proliferation and ERK1/2 upon activation of PAR2 is reversed by the metalloproteinase inhibitor batimastat, TGF-α-neutralizing antibodies, EGFR ligand binding domain-blocking antibodies, and certain EGFR tyrosine kinase inhibitors [357]. Thus, transactivation of EGFR appears to be a major mechanism whereby activation of PAR-2 results in colon cancer cell growth.

Of notice, epidermal growth factor (EGF) increases the production of MMP-7 [402]. Furthermore, some CRCs with up-regulated MMP-7 expression (activating the apoptotic activity of TGF-β) are susceptible to treatment with EGFR tyrosine kinase inhibitor (Gefitinib, Iressa™) [403].

The proliferative response to PAR-2 stimulation induces the phosphorylation of MEK1/2 and the extracellular signal-regulated kinase 1 and 2 (ERK1/2), suggesting activation of the MAPK-ERK pathway as an important function of PAR-2 in CRC [355, 357]. Similar results have been obtained in pancreatic cancer,[404] and treatment of melanoma cells with trypsin or PAR-2 agonist peptide stimulates experimental metastasis, suggesting a central role for PAR-2 in tumour invasion and metastasis [400]. Furthermore, PAR-1 (activated by thrombin) and PAR-2 is greatly overexpressed in the cells forming the tumour microenvironment (i.e. fibroblasts), suggesting that these receptors mediate the signalling of secreted thrombin and trypsin in the processes of cellular metastasis (figure 14) [405, 406]. This interesting link between trypsin, MMPs and PAR-2 in CRC progression deserves further illumination and may give way for new inhibitory targets.

TRYPSIN AND PAR-2 INDUCE PROSTAGLANDINE SYNTHESIS

In the intestines, physiological concentrations of pancreatic trypsin and a peptide corresponding to the tethered ligand of PAR-2, which is exposed by trypsin cleavage, activates a phospholipase. This causes formation of inositol trisphosphate, mobilization of Ca^{2+} and release of arachidonic acid and prostaglandins. The prostaglandins act in a paracrine and autocrine manner in the intestine to regulate epithelial transport, intestinal motility, growth, and blood flow and act to mediate inflammation and cytoprotection. Thus, trypsin is a signalling molecule that specifically regulates enterocytes by triggering PAR-2 [407].

Consequently, in addition to its role as a digestive enzyme, trypsin acts as an intestinal signalling molecule that regulates the epithelium by specifically cleaving and activating PAR-2. Theoretically, PAR-2 may propose effects on the intestinal epithelium analogue to the role of cyclooxygenase-2 (COX-2) overexpression that has been recently emphasized [311, 408, 409]. Release of prostaglandins and induction of the MAPK-ERK pathway may explain the proliferative effect of PAR-2. Recent evidence show that prostaglandin E2 (PGE$_2$) rapidly phosphorylates EGFR and triggers ERK2 mitogenic signalling in colon cancer cell lines [306]. The PGE2 transactivation of EGFR reveal a mechanism by which PGE$_2$ mediates growth of colonic polyps and cancers [306], as well as increased potential for invasion [410].

In the wake of the withdrawal of the specific COX-2 inhibitors, new inhibitory mechanisms by which colorectal adenoma development and progression can be prevented are welcomed. In this aspect, the trypsin/MMP/PAR-2 interactive play suggests a potential for future interventional therapy (figure 13). In fact, a recent animal model investigating the cooperative effect of MMP and COX-2 inhibition proved to reduce the number of intestinal adenomas at a larger scale (67% reduction of tumour multiplicity) rather than any single inhibition alone (35% for MMP alone vs. 48% for COX alone) [409]. MMP-inhibitors have so far not been subject to trials in patients with CRC, although this patient group serves as a well-recognized cancer model. Although such a theory remains to be clarified, inhibition of trypsin/PAR-2 mediated prostaglandine synthesis may pose an attractive alternative to selective COX-2 inhibition in the prevention of colorectal adenomas.

Chapter 11

CONCLUSIONS

The biological and clinical implications of molecular and preneoplastic pathways in patients with colorectal cancer are developing – development of endoscopic techniques will foster new and less invasive ways of detecting precursor lesions in the large bowel. While the adenoma-carcinoma lineage mantra has prevailed for a more than two decades, it is now established that CRC with microsatellite instability follows a pathway different from that characterized by chromosomal instability. The clinicopathological characteristics are evolving; however, the specific genetic, prognostic, and therapeutic differences remains to be clearly defined. The role of epigenetic changes, although evidently important, remains to be clearly linked to the other molecular pathways, and to clinical significance (i.e. prognostic ability, and prediction of chemotherapy response). Investigation of MSI status in CRCs is presently warranted for three reasons. First, as a potential screening tool for HNPCC; secondly, as a prognostic marker and, lastly, as a potential predictive factor of chemotherapy response. To further improve the understanding of CRC, subgroup stratification according to MSI-status appears important – as is now generally appreciated in cancer research[193]. Furthermore, the evolving understanding of the tumor microenvironment, where immune cells and protease-systems take center place, appears to hold clues to many, as of yet unanswered, key-questions in colorectal neoplasia. Prediction of disease progress and prognosis, development of new therapies, and tailoring of adjuvant therapy will likely derive through this understanding in the future.

REFERENCES

[1] Weitz J, Koch M, Debus J et al. Colorectal cancer. *Lancet.* 2005; 365: 153-165.

[2] Körner H, Søreide K, Stokkeland PJ, Søreide JA. Systematic Follow-up After Curative Surgery for Colorectal Cancer in Norway: A Population-Based Audit of Effectiveness, Costs, and Compliance. *J. Gastrointest. Surg.* 2005; 9: 320-328.

[3] Körner H, Søreide K, Stokkeland PJ, Søreide JA. Diagnostic Accuracy of Serum-Carcino-embryonic Antigen in Recurrent Colorectal Cancer: A Receiver Operating Characteristics Curve Analysis. *Ann. Surg. Oncol.* 2006 in press.

[4] Søreide K, Janssen EA, Søiland H et al. Microsatellite instability in colorectal cancer. *Br. J. Surg.* 2006; 93: 395-406.

[5] Gervaz P, Bucher P, Morel P. Two colons-two cancers: paradigm shift and clinical implications. *J. Surg. Oncol.* 2004; 88: 261-266.

[6] Gervaz P, Cerottini JP, Bouzourene H et al. Comparison of microsatellite instability and chromosomal instability in predicting survival of patients with T3N0 colorectal cancer. *Surgery.* 2002; 131: 190-197.

[7] Haydon AM, Jass JR. Emerging pathways in colorectal-cancer development. *Lancet Oncol.* 2002; 3: 83-88.

[8] Jass JR, Whitehall VL, Young J, Leggett BA. Emerging concepts in colorectal neoplasia. *Gastroenterology.* 2002; 123: 862-876.

[9] Jass JR, Young J, Leggett BA. Evolution of colorectal cancer: change of pace and change of direction. *J. Gastroenterol. Hepatol.* 2002; 17: 17-26.

[10] Sugai T, Habano W, Jiao YF et al. Analysis of allelic imbalances at multiple cancer-related chromosomal loci and microsatellite instability within the same tumor using a single tumor gland from colorectal carcinomas. *Int. J. Cancer.* 2005; 114: 337-345.

[11] Gryfe R, Kim H, Hsieh ET et al. Tumor microsatellite instability and clinical outcome in young patients with colorectal cancer. *N. Engl. J. Med.* 2000; 342: 69-77.

[12] Kohonen-Corish MR, Daniel JJ, Chan C et al. Low microsatellite instability is associated with poor prognosis in stage C colon cancer. *J. Clin. Oncol.* 2005; 23: 2318-2324.

[13] Popat S, Hubner R, Houlston RS. Systematic review of microsatellite instability and colorectal cancer prognosis. *J. Clin. Oncol.* 2005; 23: 609-618.

[14] Ribic CM, Sargent DJ, Moore MJ et al. Tumor microsatellite-instability status as a predictor of benefit from fluorouracil-based adjuvant chemotherapy for colon cancer. *N. Engl. J. Med.* 2003; 349: 247-257.

[15] Wright CM, Dent OF, Newland RC et al. Low level microsatellite instability may be associated with reduced cancer specific survival in sporadic stage C colorectal carcinoma. *Gut.* 2005; 54: 103-108.

[16] Anwar S, Frayling IM, Scott NA, Carlson GL. Systematic review of genetic influences on the prognosis of colorectal cancer. *Br. J. Surg.* 2004; 91: 1275-1291.

[17] Koornstra JJ, de Jong S, Hollema H et al. Changes in apoptosis during the development of colorectal cancer: a systematic review of the literature. *Crit. Rev. Oncol. Hematol.* 2003; 45: 37-53.

[18] Munro AJ, Lain S, Lane DP. P53 abnormalities and outcomes in colorectal cancer: a systematic review. *Br. J. Cancer.* 2005; 92: 434-444.

[19] Popat S, Matakidou A, Houlston RS. Thymidylate synthase expression and prognosis in colorectal cancer: a systematic review and meta-analysis. *J. Clin. Oncol.* 2004; 22: 529-536.

[20] Søreide K, Janssen E, Kørner H, Baak J. Trypsin in colorectal cancer: molecular biological mechanisms of proliferation, invasion, and metastasis. *J. Pathol.* 2006; 209: 147-156.

[21] Hahn WC, Weinberg RA. Rules for making human tumor cells. *N. Engl. J. Med.* 2002; 347: 1593-1603.

[22] Hanahan D, Weinberg RA. The hallmarks of cancer. *Cell* 2000; 100: 57-70.

[23] Fearon ER, Vogelstein B. A genetic model for colorectal tumorigenesis. *Cell.* 1990; 61: 759-767.

[24] Huang J, Papadopoulos N, McKinley AJ et al. APC mutations in colorectal tumors with mismatch repair deficiency. *Proc. Natl. Acad. Sci. U. S. A.* 1996; 93: 9049-9054.

[25] Kinzler KW, Vogelstein B. Lessons from hereditary colorectal cancer. *Cell.* 1996; 87: 159-170.

[26] Lengauer C, Kinzler KW, Vogelstein B. DNA methylation and genetic instability in colorectal cancer cells. *Proc. Natl. Acad. Sci. U. S. A.* 1997; 94: 2545-2550.

[27] Liu B, Parsons R, Papadopoulos N et al. Analysis of mismatch repair genes in hereditary non-polyposis colorectal cancer patients. *Nat. Med.* 1996; 2: 169-174.

[28] Parsons R, Li GM, Longley MJ et al. Hypermutability and mismatch repair deficiency in RER+ tumor cells. *Cell.* 1993; 75: 1227-1236.

[29] Smith G, Carey FA, Beattie J et al. Mutations in APC, Kirsten-ras, and p53--alternative genetic pathways to colorectal cancer. *Proc. Natl. Acad. Sci. U. S. A.* 2002; 99: 9433-9438.

[30] Leslie A, Pratt NR, Gillespie K et al. Mutations of APC, K-ras, and p53 are associated with specific chromosomal aberrations in colorectal adenocarcinomas. *Cancer Res.* 2003; 63: 4656-4661.

[31] Conlin A, Smith G, Carey FA et al. The prognostic significance of K-ras, p53, and APC mutations in colorectal carcinoma. *Gut.* 2005; 54: 1283-1286.

[32] Loeb LA, Loeb KR, Anderson JP. Multiple mutations and cancer. *Proc. Natl. Acad. Sci. U. S. A.* 2003; 100: 776-781.

[33] Loeb LA. A mutator phenotype in cancer. *Cancer Res.* 2001; 61: 3230-3239.

[34] Choi SW, Lee KJ, Bae YA et al. Genetic classification of colorectal cancer based on chromosomal loss and microsatellite instability predicts survival. *Clin. Cancer Res.* 2002; 8: 2311-2322.

[35] Giaretti W, Rapallo A, Sciutto A et al. Intratumor heterogeneity of k-ras and p53 mutations among human colorectal adenomas containing early cancer. *Anal. Cell Pathol.* 2000; 21: 49-57.

[36] Hermsen M, Postma C, Baak J et al. Colorectal adenoma to carcinoma progression follows multiple pathways of chromosomal instability. *Gastroenterology.* 2002; 123: 1109-1119.

[37] Kennedy EP, Hamilton SR. Genetics of colorectal cancer. *Semin. Surg. Oncol.* 1998; 15: 126-130.

[38] Liu B, Farrington SM, Petersen GM et al. Genetic instability occurs in the majority of young patients with colorectal cancer. *Nat. Med.* 1995; 1: 348-352.

[39] Meijer GA, Hermsen MA, Baak JP et al. Progression from colorectal adenoma to carcinoma is associated with non-random chromosomal gains as detected by comparative genomic hybridisation. *J. Clin. Pathol.* 1998; 51: 901-909.

[40] Postma C, Hermsen MA, Coffa J et al. Chromosomal instability in flat adenomas and carcinomas of the colon. *J. Pathol.* 2005; 205: 514-521.

[41] Aquilina G, Hess P, Branch P et al. A mismatch recognition defect in colon carcinoma confers DNA microsatellite instability and a mutator phenotype. *Proc. Natl. Acad. Sci. U. S. A.* 1994; 91: 8905-8909.

[42] Jass JR, Cottier DS, Jeevaratnam P et al. Diagnostic use of microsatellite instability in hereditary non-polyposis colorectal cancer. *Lancet.* 1995; 346: 1200-1201.

[43] Perucho M. Microsatellite instability: the mutator that mutates the other mutator. *Nat. Med.* 1996; 2: 630-631.

[44] Thibodeau SN, Bren G, Schaid D. Microsatellite instability in cancer of the proximal colon. *Science.* 1993; 260: 816-819.

[45] Merg A, Lynch HT, Lynch JF, Howe JR. Hereditary colorectal cancer-part II. *Curr. Probl. Surg.* 2005; 42: 267-333.

[46] Merg A, Lynch HT, Lynch JF, Howe JR. Hereditary colon cancer--part I. *Curr. Probl. Surg.* 2005; 42: 195-256.

[47] de la Chapelle A. Microsatellite instability. *N. Engl. J. Med.* 2003; 349: 209-210.

[48] Lynch HT, de la Chapelle A. Hereditary colorectal cancer. *N. Engl. J. Med.* 2003; 348: 919-932.

[49] Chung DC, Rustgi AK. The hereditary nonpolyposis colorectal cancer syndrome: genetics and clinical implications. *Ann. Intern. Med.* 2003; 138: 560-570.

[50] Aaltonen LA, Peltomaki P, Mecklin JP et al. Replication errors in benign and malignant tumors from hereditary nonpolyposis colorectal cancer patients. *Cancer Res.* 1994; 54: 1645-1648.

[51] Cunningham JM, Christensen ER, Tester DJ et al. Hypermethylation of the hMLH1 promoter in colon cancer with microsatellite instability. *Cancer Res.* 1998; 58: 3455-3460.

[52] Umar A, Boland CR, Terdiman JP et al. Revised Bethesda Guidelines for hereditary nonpolyposis colorectal cancer (Lynch syndrome) and microsatellite instability. *J. Natl. Cancer Inst.* 2004; 96: 261-268.

[53] Boland CR, Thibodeau SN, Hamilton SR et al. A National Cancer Institute Workshop on Microsatellite Instability for cancer detection and familial predisposition: development of international criteria for the determination of microsatellite instability in colorectal cancer. *Cancer Res.* 1998; 58: 5248-5257.

[54] Pinol V, Castells A, Andreu M et al. Accuracy of revised Bethesda guidelines, microsatellite instability, and immunohistochemistry for the identification of patients with hereditary nonpolyposis colorectal cancer. *JAMA.* 2005; 293: 1986-1994.

[55] Lynch HT, Lynch PM. Molecular screening for the Lynch syndrome--better than family history? *N. Engl. J. Med.* 2005; 352: 1920-1922.

[56] Hampel H, Frankel WL, Martin E et al. Screening for the Lynch syndrome (hereditary nonpolyposis colorectal cancer). *N. Engl. J. Med.* 2005; 352: 1851-1860.

[57] Bouzourene H, Taminelli L, Chaubert P et al. A cost-effective algorithm for hereditary nonpolyposis colorectal cancer detection. *Am. J. Clin. Pathol.* 2006; 125: 823-831.

[58] Boland CR. Decoding hereditary colorectal cancer. *N. Engl. J. Med.* 2006; 354: 2815-2817.

[59] Matsumoto T, Iida M, Kobori Y et al. Serrated adenoma in familial adenomatous polyposis: relation to germline APC gene mutation. *Gut.* 2002; 50: 402-404.

[60] Powell SM, Zilz N, Beazer-Barclay Y et al. APC mutations occur early during colorectal tumorigenesis. *Nature.* 1992; 359: 235-237.

[61] Oshima M, Oshima H, Kitagawa K et al. Loss of Apc heterozygosity and abnormal tissue building in nascent intestinal polyps in mice carrying a truncated Apc gene. *Proc. Natl. Acad. Sci. U. S. A.* 1995; 92: 4482-4486.

[62] Schottenfeld D, Beebe-Dimmer J. Chronic inflammation: a common and important factor in the pathogenesis of neoplasia. *CA Cancer J. Clin.* 2006; 56: 69-83.

[63] van Kempen LC, de Visser KE, Coussens LM. Inflammation, proteases and cancer. *Eur. J. Cancer.* 2006; 42: 728-734.

[64] Clevers H. At the crossroads of inflammation and cancer. *Cell.* 2004; 118: 671-674.

[65] Coussens LM, Werb Z. Inflammation and cancer. *Nature.* 2002; 420: 860-867.

[66] Balkwill F, Mantovani A. Inflammation and cancer: back to Virchow? *Lancet.* 2001; 357: 539-545.

[67] Dvorak HF. Tumors: wounds that do not heal. Similarities between tumor stroma generation and wound healing. *N. Engl. J. Med.* 1986; 315: 1650-1659.

[68] Pages F, Berger A, Camus M et al. Effector memory T cells, early metastasis, and survival in colorectal cancer. *N. Engl. J. Med.* 2005; 353: 2654-2666.

[69] Wikstrom K, Ohd JF, Sjolander A. Regulation of leukotriene-dependent induction of cyclooxygenase-2 and Bcl-2. *Biochem. Biophys. Res. Commun.* 2003; 302: 330-335.

[70] Sheng H, Shao J, Washington MK, DuBois RN. Prostaglandin E2 increases growth and motility of colorectal carcinoma cells. *J. Biol. Chem.* 2001; 276: 18075-18081.

[71] Tsujii M, Kawano S, DuBois RN. Cyclooxygenase-2 expression in human colon cancer cells increases metastatic potential. *Proc. Natl. Acad. Sci. U. S. A.* 1997; 94: 3336-3340.

[72] Poligone B, Baldwin AS. Positive and negative regulation of NF-kappaB by COX-2: roles of different prostaglandins. *J. Biol. Chem.* 2001; 276: 38658-38664.

[73] Ruegg C. Leukocytes, inflammation, and angiogenesis in cancer: fatal attractions. *J. Leukoc. Biol.* 2006.

[74] DuBois RN. Leukotriene A4 signaling, inflammation, and cancer. *J. Natl. Cancer Inst.* 2003; 95: 1028-1029.

[75] van der Woude CJ, Kleibeuker JH, Jansen PL, Moshage H. Chronic inflammation, apoptosis and (pre-)malignant lesions in the gastro-intestinal tract. *Apoptosis.* 2004; 9: 123-130.

[76] Ekbom A, Helmick C, Zack M, Adami HO. Ulcerative colitis and colorectal cancer. A population-based study. *N. Engl. J. Med.* 1990; 323: 1228-1233.

[77] Itzkowitz SH, Yio X. Inflammation and cancer IV. Colorectal cancer in inflammatory bowel disease: the role of inflammation. *Am. J. Physiol. Gastrointest. Liver Physiol.* 2004; 287: G7-17.

[78] Rhodes JM, Campbell BJ. Inflammation and colorectal cancer: IBD-associated and sporadic cancer compared. *Trends Mol. Med.* 2002; 8: 10-16.

[79] Delaunoit T, Limburg PJ, Goldberg RM et al. Colorectal cancer prognosis among patients with inflammatory bowel disease. *Clin. Gastroenterol. Hepatol.* 2006; 4: 335-342.

[80] Vagefi PA, Longo WE. Colorectal cancer in patients with inflammatory bowel disease. *Clin. Colorectal Cancer.* 2005; 4: 313-319.

[81] Vera A, Gunson BK, Ussatoff V et al. Colorectal cancer in patients with inflammatory bowel disease after liver transplantation for primary sclerosing cholangitis. *Transplantation.* 2003; 75: 1983-1988.

[82] Murthy S, Flanigan A, Clearfield H. Colorectal cancer in inflammatory bowel disease: molecular and clinical features. *Gastroenterol. Clin. North Am.* 2002; 31: 551-564, x.

[83] Mayer R, Wong WD, Rothenberger DA et al. Colorectal cancer in inflammatory bowel disease: a continuing problem. *Dis. Colon. Rectum.* 1999; 42: 343-347.

[84] Fonager K, Sorensen HT, Mellemkjaer L et al. Risk of colorectal cancer in relatives of patients with inflammatory bowel disease (Denmark). *Cancer Causes Control.* 1998; 9: 389-392.

[85] Delpre G, Kadish U. A genetic predisposition for colorectal cancer in inflammatory bowel disease. *Gut.* 1988; 29: 1618.

[86] Hofseth LJ, Khan MA, Ambrose M et al. The adaptive imbalance in base excision-repair enzymes generates microsatellite instability in chronic inflammation. *J. Clin. Invest.* 2003; 112: 1887-1894.

[87] Guo HH, Loeb LA. Tumbling down a different pathway to genetic instability. *J. Clin. Invest.* 2003; 112: 1793-1795.

[88] Nguyen C, Coelho AM, Grady E et al. Colitis induced by proteinase-activated receptor-2 agonists is mediated by a neurogenic mechanism. *Can. J. Physiol. Pharmacol.* 2003; 81: 920-927.

[89] Jaiswal M, LaRusso NF, Gores GJ. Nitric oxide in gastrointestinal epithelial cell carcinogenesis: linking inflammation to oncogenesis. *Am. J. Physiol. Gastrointest. Liver Physiol.* 2001; 281: G626-634.

[90] Boland CR, Luciani MG, Gasche C, Goel A. Infection, inflammation, and gastrointestinal cancer. *Gut.* 2005; 54: 1321-1331.

[91] Karin M. Inflammation and cancer: the long reach of Ras. *Nat. Med.* 2005; 11: 20-21.

[92] Pikarsky E, Porat RM, Stein I et al. NF-kappaB functions as a tumour promoter in inflammation-associated cancer. *Nature.* 2004; 431: 461-466.

[93] Greten FR, Eckmann L, Greten TF et al. IKKbeta links inflammation and tumorigenesis in a mouse model of colitis-associated cancer. *Cell.* 2004; 118: 285-296.

[94] Wielockx B, Libert C, Wilson C. Matrilysin (matrix metalloproteinase-7): a new promising drug target in cancer and inflammation? *Cytokine Growth Factor Rev.* 2004; 15: 111-115.

[95] Macarthur M, Hold GL, El-Omar EM. Inflammation and Cancer II. Role of chronic inflammation and cytokine gene polymorphisms in the pathogenesis of gastrointestinal malignancy. *Am. J. Physiol. Gastrointest. Liver Physiol.* 2004; 286: G515-520.

[96] Weaver SA, Ward SG. Phosphoinositide 3-kinases in the gut: a link between inflammation and cancer? *Trends Mol. Med.* 2001; 7: 455-462.

[97] Eaden JA, Mayberry JF. Guidelines for screening and surveillance of asymptomatic colorectal cancer in patients with inflammatory bowel disease. *Gut.* 2002; 51 Suppl 5: V10-12.

[98] Lashner BA. Colorectal cancer surveillance for patients with inflammatory bowel disease. *Gastrointest Endosc. Clin. N. Am.* 2002; 12: 135-143, viii.

[99] Collins PD, Mpofu C, Watson AJ, Rhodes JM. Strategies for detecting colon cancer and/or dysplasia in patients with inflammatory bowel disease. *Cochrane Database Syst. Rev.* 2006; CD000279.

[100] Rubin DT. The changing face of colorectal cancer in inflammatory bowel disease: progress at last! *Gastroenterology.* 2006; 130: 1350-1352.

[101] Jess T, Loftus EV, Jr., Velayos FS et al. Risk of intestinal cancer in inflammatory bowel disease: a population-based study from olmsted county, Minnesota. *Gastroenterology.* 2006; 130: 1039-1046.

[102] Rutter MD, Saunders BP, Wilkinson KH et al. Thirty-year analysis of a colonoscopic surveillance program for neoplasia in ulcerative colitis. *Gastroenterology.* 2006; 130: 1030-1038.

[103] Hoff G, Bretthauer M. The *science* and politics of colorectal cancer screening. *PLoS. Med.* 2006; 3: e36; quiz e104.

[104] Recommendation to include colorectal cancer screening in public health policy. The European Group for Colorectal Cancer Screening. *J. Med. Screen.* 1999; 6: 80-81.

[105] Kronborg O, Fenger C, Olsen J et al. Randomised study of screening for colorectal cancer with faecal-occult-blood test. *Lancet.* 1996; 348: 1467-1471.

[106] Ransohoff DF, Sandler RS. Clinical practice. Screening for colorectal cancer. *N. Engl. J. Med.* 2002; 346: 40-44.

[107] Lieberman DA, Weiss DG. One-time screening for colorectal cancer with combined fecal occult-blood testing and examination of the distal colon. *N. Engl. J. Med.* 2001; 345: 555-560.

[108] Allison JE, Tekawa IS, Ransom LJ, Adrain AL. A comparison of fecal occult-blood tests for colorectal-cancer screening. *N. Engl. J. Med.* 1996; 334: 155-159.

[109] Dubois G. Screening for colorectal cancer. French Working Group on Colorectal Cancer Screening. *N. Engl. J. Med.* 1995; 333: 460-461.

[110] Mandel JS, Bond JH, Church TR et al. Reducing mortality from colorectal cancer by screening for fecal occult blood. Minnesota Colon Cancer Control Study. *N. Engl. J. Med.* 1993; 328: 1365-1371.

[111] Selby JV, Friedman GD, Quesenberry CP, Jr., Weiss NS. A case-control study of screening sigmoidoscopy and mortality from colorectal cancer. *N. Engl. J. Med.* 1992; 326: 653-657.

[112] Hurlstone DP, Karajeh MA, Shorthouse AJ. Screening for colorectal cancer: implications for UK and European initiatives. *Tech. Coloproctol.* 2004; 8: 139-145.

[113] Woolf SH. A smarter strategy? Reflections on fecal DNA screening for colorectal cancer. *N. Engl. J. Med.* 2004; 351: 2755-2758.

[114] Imperiale TF, Ransohoff DF, Itzkowitz SH et al. Fecal DNA versus fecal occult blood for colorectal-cancer screening in an average-risk population. *N. Engl. J. Med.* 2004; 351: 2704-2714.

[115] Muto T, Nagawa H, Watanabe T et al. Colorectal carcinogenesis: historical review. *Dis. Colon. Rectum.* 1997; 40: S80-85.

[116] Konishi M, Kikuchi-Yanoshita R, Tanaka K et al. Molecular *nature* of colon tumors in hereditary nonpolyposis colon cancer, familial polyposis, and sporadic colon cancer. *Gastroenterology.* 1996; 111: 307-317.

[117] Vogelstein B, Fearon ER, Hamilton SR et al. Genetic alterations during colorectal-tumor development. *N. Engl. J. Med.* 1988; 319: 525-532.

[118] Bedenne L, Faivre J, Boutron MC et al. Adenoma--carcinoma sequence or "de novo" carcinogenesis? A study of adenomatous remnants in a population-based series of large bowel cancers. *Cancer.* 1992; 69: 883-888.

[119] Kudo S, Tamura S, Hirota S et al. The problem of de novo colorectal carcinoma. *Eur. J. Cancer.* 1995; 31A: 1118-1120.

[120] Shimoda T, Ikegami M, Fujisaki J et al. Early colorectal carcinoma with special reference to its development de novo. *Cancer.* 1989; 64: 1138-1146.

[121] Hermanek P, Gall FP. Early (microinvasive) colorectal carcinoma. Pathology, diagnosis, surgical treatment. *Int. J. Colorectal. Dis.* 1986; 1: 79-84.

[122] Mueller JD, Bethke B, Stolte M. Colorectal de novo carcinoma: a review of its diagnosis, histopathology, molecular biology, and clinical relevance. *Virchows. Arch.* 2002; 440: 453-460.

[123] Jass J, Sobin L. Histological typing of intestinal tumors. In organization WH (ed) Edition 2nd edition. Springer-Verlag 1992.
[124] Schlemper RJ, Itabashi M, Kato Y et al. Differences in the diagnostic criteria used by Japanese and Western pathologists to diagnose colorectal carcinoma. *Cancer.* 1998; 82: 60-69.
[125] Schlemper RJ, Riddell RH, Kato Y et al. The Vienna classification of gastrointestinal epithelial neoplasia. *Gut.* 2000; 47: 251-255.
[126] Luo L, Shen GQ, Stiffler KA et al. Loss of heterozygosity in human aberrant crypt foci (ACF), a putative precursor of colon cancer. *Carcinogenesis.* 2006; 27: 1153-1159.
[127] Rudolph RE, Dominitz JA, Lampe JW et al. Risk factors for colorectal cancer in relation to number and size of aberrant crypt foci in humans. *Cancer Epidemiol. Biomarkers Prev.* 2005; 14: 605-608.
[128] Nascimbeni R, Villanacci V, Mariani PP et al. Aberrant crypt foci in the human colon: frequency and histologic patterns in patients with colorectal cancer or diverticular disease. *Am. J. Surg. Pathol.* 1999; 23: 1256-1263.
[129] Takayama T, Katsuki S, Takahashi Y et al. Aberrant crypt foci of the colon as precursors of adenoma and cancer. *N. Engl. J. Med.* 1998; 339: 1277-1284.
[130] Alrawi SJ, Schiff M, Carroll RE et al. Aberrant crypt foci. *Anticancer Res.* 2006; 26: 107-119.
[131] Nambiar PR, Nakanishi M, Gupta R et al. Genetic signatures of high- and low-risk aberrant crypt foci in a mouse model of sporadic colon cancer. *Cancer Res.* 2004; 64: 6394-6401.
[132] Kudo S, Hirota S, Nakajima T et al. Colorectal tumours and pit pattern. *J. Clin. Pathol.* 1994; 47: 880-885.
[133] Pretlow TP, Pretlow TG. Mutant KRAS in aberrant crypt foci (ACF): initiation of colorectal cancer? *Biochim. Biophys. Acta.* 2005; 1756: 83-96.
[134] Takayama T, Ohi M, Hayashi T et al. Analysis of K-ras, APC, and beta-catenin in aberrant crypt foci in sporadic adenoma, cancer, and familial adenomatous polyposis. *Gastroenterology.* 2001; 121: 599-611.
[135] Cohen G, Mustafi R, Chumsangsri A et al. Epidermal growth factor receptor signaling is up-regulated in human colonic aberrant crypt foci. *Cancer Res.* 2006; 66: 5656-5664.
[136] Goldstein NS. Serrated pathway and APC (conventional)-type colorectal polyps: molecular-morphologic correlations, genetic pathways, and implications for classification. *Am. J. Clin. Pathol.* 2006; 125: 146-153.

[137] Hurlstone DP, Karajeh M, Sanders DS et al. Rectal aberrant crypt foci identified using high-magnification-chromoscopic colonoscopy: biomarkers for flat and depressed neoplasia. *Am. J. Gastroenterol.* 2005; 100: 1283-1289.

[138] Scheiden R, Sand J, Pandin M et al. Colorectal high-grade adenomas: incidence, localization and adenoma-adenocarcinoma ratio in a retrospective and comparative population-based study of 225 consecutive cases between 1988 and 1996. *Int. J. Colorectal Dis.* 2000; 15: 29-34.

[139] Giacosa A, Frascio F, Munizzi F. Epidemiology of colorectal polyps. *Tech. Coloproctol.* 2004; 8 Suppl 2: s243-247.

[140] Kariya J, Mizuno K, Mayama M. A case of early colorectal cancer type IIc associated with familial polyposis coli. *Stomach intestine.* 1977; 12: 1359-1364 (in Japanese with English abstract).

[141] Tsuda S, Veress B, Toth E, Fork FT. Flat and depressed colorectal tumours in a southern Swedish population: a prospective chromoendoscopic and histopathological study. *Gut.* 2002; 51: 550-555.

[142] Haggitt RC, Glotzbach RE, Soffer EE, Wruble LD. Prognostic factors in colorectal carcinomas arising in adenomas: implications for lesions removed by endoscopic polypectomy. *Gastroenterology.* 1985; 89: 328-336.

[143] Kudo S, Kashida H, Tamura T et al. Colonoscopic diagnosis and management of nonpolypoid early colorectal cancer. *World J. Surg.* 2000; 24: 1081-1090.

[144] Kashida H, Kudo SE. Early colorectal cancer: concept, diagnosis, and management. *Int J. Clin. Oncol.* 2006; 11: 1-8.

[145] Kudo S, Kashida H, Tamura S, Nakajima T. The problem of "flat" colonic adenoma. *Gastrointest Endosc. Clin. N. Am.* 1997; 7: 87-98.

[146] Kudo S, Kashida H, Nakajima T et al. Endoscopic diagnosis and treatment of early colorectal cancer. *World J. Surg.* 1997; 21: 694-701.

[147] Kudo S, Kashida H, Tamura T. Early colorectal cancer: flat or depressed type. *J. Gastroenterol. Hepatol.* 2000; 15 Suppl: D66-70.

[148] Kudo S, Tamura S, Nakajima T et al. Diagnosis of colorectal tumorous lesions by magnifying endoscopy. *Gastrointest. Endosc.* 1996; 44: 8-14.

[149] Kudo S. Endoscopic mucosal resection of flat and depressed types of early colorectal cancer. *Endoscopy.* 1993; 25: 455-461.

[150] de Graaf EJ. Transanal endoscopic micro*surgery*. *Scand. J. Gastroenterol. Suppl.* 2003; 34-39.

[151] Ganai S, Kanumuri P, Rao RS, Alexander AI. Local recurrence after transanal endoscopic micro*surgery* for rectal polyps and early cancers. *Ann. Surg. Oncol.* 2006; 13: 547-556.

[152] Guerrieri M, Baldarelli M, Morino M et al. Transanal endoscopic micro*surgery* in rectal adenomas: experience of six Italian centres. *Dig. Liver Dis.* 2006; 38: 202-207.

[153] Middleton PF, Sutherland LM, Maddern GJ. Transanal endoscopic micro*surgery*: a systematic review. *Dis. Colon. Rectum.* 2005; 48: 270-284.

[154] Søreide K, Immervoll H, Molven A. Precursors to pancreatic cancer. *Tidsskr. Nor. Laegeforen.* 2006; 126: 905-908.

[155] Søreide K, Gudlaugsson E, Kjellevold KH. Appendiceal mucinous cystadenoma. *Tidsskr. Nor. Laegeforen.* 2005; 125: 289-291.

[156] Bhanot U, Heydrich R, Moller P, Hasel C. Survivin expression in pancreatic intraepithelial neoplasia (PanIN): steady increase along the developmental stages of pancreatic ductal adenocarcinoma. *Am. J. Surg. Pathol.* 2006; 30: 754-759.

[157] Behrens A, May A, Gossner L et al. Curative treatment for high-grade intraepithelial neoplasia in Barrett's esophagus. *Endoscopy.* 2005; 37: 999-1005.

[158] Takaori K, Hruban RH, Maitra A, Tanigawa N. Pancreatic intraepithelial neoplasia. *Pancreas.* 2004; 28: 257-262.

[159] Hruban RH, Takaori K, Klimstra DS et al. An illustrated consensus on the classification of pancreatic intraepithelial neoplasia and intraductal papillary mucinous neoplasms. *Am. J. Surg. Pathol.* 2004; 28: 977-987.

[160] Kirchner T, Muller S, Hattori T et al. Metaplasia, intraepithelial neoplasia and early cancer of the stomach are related to dedifferentiated epithelial cells defined by cytokeratin-7 expression in gastritis. *Virchows Arch.* 2001; 439: 512-522.

[161] Hecht JL, Ince TA, Baak JP et al. Prediction of endometrial carcinoma by subjective endometrial intraepithelial neoplasia diagnosis. *Mod. Pathol.* 2005; 18: 324-330.

[162] Baak JP, Mutter GL, Robboy S et al. The molecular genetics and morphometry-based endometrial intraepithelial neoplasia classification system predicts disease progression in endometrial hyperplasia more accurately than the 1994 World Health Organization classification system. *Cancer.* 2005; 103: 2304-2312.

[163] Baak JP, Mutter GL. EIN and WHO94. *J. Clin. Pathol.* 2005; 58: 1-6.

[164] Baak JP, Kruse AJ, Robboy SJ et al. Dynamic behavioural interpretation of cervical intraepithelial neoplasia (CIN) by molecular biomarkers. *J. Clin. Pathol.* 2006.

[165] Baak JP, Kruse AJ. Use of biomarkers in the evaluation of CIN grade and progression of early CIN. *Methods Mol. Med.* 2005; 119: 85-99.

[166] Schoen RE. The case for population-based screening for colorectal cancer. *Nat. Rev. Cancer.* 2002; 2: 65-70.

[167] Winawer SJ. Screening of colorectal cancer: progress and problems. Recent Results. *Cancer Res.* 2005; 166: 231-244.

[168] Kelloff GJ, Lippman SM, Dannenberg AJ et al. Progress in chemoprevention drug development: the promise of molecular biomarkers for prevention of intraepithelial neoplasia and cancer--a plan to move forward. *Clin. Cancer Res.* 2006; 12: 3661-3697.

[169] Srivastava S, Verma M, Henson DE. Biomarkers for early detection of colon cancer. *Clin. Cancer Res.* 2001; 7: 1118-1126.

[170] Winawer SJ. Screening of colorectal cancer. *Surg. Oncol. Clin. N. Am.* 2005; 14: 699-722.

[171] Søreide K, Buter TC, Janssen E et al. A monotonous population of elongated cells (MPECs) identifies colorectal adenomas at high risk of metachronous cancer. *Am. J. Surg. Pathol.* 2006, September issue, in press.

[172] Søreide K, Buter TC, Janssen E et al. *Cell cycle, apoptosis markers and MPECs in colorectal adenoma predict metachronous cancer development.* Submitted 2006.

[173] Furlan D, Casati B, Cerutti R et al. Genetic progression in sporadic endometrial and gastrointestinal cancers with high microsatellite instability. *J. Pathol.* 2002; 197: 603-609.

[174] Kim IJ, Kang HC, Park JH et al. Development and applications of a beta-catenin oligonucleotide microarray: beta-catenin mutations are dominantly found in the proximal colon cancers with microsatellite instability. *Clin Cancer Res.* 2003; 9: 2920-2925.

[175] Samowitz WS, Holden JA, Curtin K et al. Inverse relationship between microsatellite instability and K-ras and p53 gene alterations in colon cancer. *Am. J. Pathol.* 2001; 158: 1517-1524.

[176] Fernandez-Peralta AM, Nejda N, Oliart S et al. Significance of mutations in TGFBR2 and BAX in neoplastic progression and patient outcome in sporadic colorectal tumors with high-frequency microsatellite instability. *Cancer Genet Cytogenet.* 2005; 157: 18-24.

[177] Giatromanolaki A, Sivridis E, Stathopoulos GP et al. Bax protein expression in colorectal cancer: association with p53, bcl-2 and patterns of relapse. *Anticancer Res.* 2001; 21: 253-259.

[178] Jansson A, Sun XF. Bax expression decreases significantly from primary tumor to metastasis in colorectal cancer. *J. Clin. Oncol.* 2002; 20: 811-816.

[179] Katsumata K, Sumi T, Tomioka H et al. Induction of apoptosis by p53, bax, bcl-2, and p21 expressed in colorectal cancer. *Int. J. Clin. Oncol.* 2003; 8: 352-356.

[180] Trojan J, Brieger A, Raedle J et al. BAX and caspase-5 frameshift mutations and spontaneous apoptosis in colorectal cancer with microsatellite instability. *Int. J. Colorectal. Dis.* 2004; 19: 538-544.

[181] Mandal M, Adam L, Mendelsohn J, Kumar R. Nuclear targeting of Bax during apoptosis in human colorectal cancer cells. *Oncogene.* 1998; 17: 999-1007.

[182] Sturm I, Kohne CH, Wolff G et al. Analysis of the p53/BAX pathway in colorectal cancer: low BAX is a negative prognostic factor in patients with resected liver metastases. *J. Clin. Oncol.* 1999; 17: 1364-1374.

[183] Markowitz S, Wang J, Myeroff L et al. Inactivation of the type II TGF-beta receptor in colon cancer cells with microsatellite instability. *Science.* 1995; 268: 1336-1338.

[184] Chen ML, Pittet MJ, Gorelik L et al. Regulatory T cells suppress tumor-specific CD8 T cell cytotoxicity through TGF-beta signals in vivo. *Proc. Natl. Acad. Sci. U. S. A.* 2005; 102: 419-424.

[185] Fink SP, Mikkola D, Willson JK, Markowitz S. TGF-beta-induced nuclear localization of Smad2 and Smad3 in Smad4 null cancer cell lines. *Oncogene.* 2003; 22: 1317-1323.

[186] Fukushima T, Mashiko M, Takita K et al. Mutational analysis of TGF-beta type II receptor, Smad2, Smad3, Smad4, Smad6 and Smad7 genes in colorectal cancer. *J. Exp. Clin. Cancer Res.* 2003; 22: 315-320.

[187] Li F, Cao Y, Townsend CM, Jr., Ko TC. TGF-beta signaling in colon cancer cells. *World J. Surg.* 2005; 29: 306-311.

[188] Roberts AB, Wakefield LM. The two faces of transforming growth factor beta in carcinogenesis. *Proc. Natl. Acad. Sci. U. S. A.* 2003; 100: 8621-8623.

[189] Banerjea A, Ahmed S, Hands RE et al. Colorectal cancers with microsatellite instability display mRNA expression signatures characteristic of increased immunogenicity. *Mol. Cancer.* 2004; 3: 21.

[190] Goel A, Arnold CN, Niedzwiecki D et al. Frequent inactivation of PTEN by promoter hypermethylation in microsatellite instability-high sporadic colorectal cancers. *Cancer Res.* 2004; 64: 3014-3021.
[191] Kim H, Nam SW, Rhee H et al. Different gene expression profiles between microsatellite instability-high and microsatellite stable colorectal carcinomas. *Oncogene.* 2004; 23: 6218-6225.
[192] Mori Y, Yin J, Sato F et al. Identification of genes uniquely involved in frequent microsatellite instability colon carcinogenesis by expression profiling combined with epigenetic scanning. *Cancer Res.* 2004; 64: 2434-2438.
[193] Baak JPA, Janssen EAM, Søreide K, Heikillae R. Genomics and proteomics - the way forward. *Ann. Oncol.* 2005; (Supplement 2): ii30-ii44.
[194] Mori S, Ogata Y, Shirouzu K. Biological features of sporadic colorectal carcinoma with high-frequency microsatellite instability: special reference to tumor proliferation and apoptosis. *Int. J. Clin. Oncol.* 2004; 9: 322-329.
[195] Prall F, Duhrkop T, Weirich V et al. Prognostic role of CD8+ tumor-infiltrating lymphocytes in stage III colorectal cancer with and without microsatellite instability. *Hum. Pathol.* 2004; 35: 808-816.
[196] Raut CP, Pawlik TM, Rodriguez-Bigas MA. Clinicopathologic features in colorectal cancer patients with microsatellite instability. *Mutat. Res.* 2004; 568: 275-282.
[197] Young J, Simms LA, Biden KG et al. Features of colorectal cancers with high-level microsatellite instability occurring in familial and sporadic settings: parallel pathways of tumorigenesis. *Am. J. Pathol.* 2001; 159: 2107-2116.
[198] Phillips SM, Banerjea A, Feakins R et al. Tumour-infiltrating lymphocytes in colorectal cancer with microsatellite instability are activated and cytotoxic. *Br. J. Surg.* 2004; 91: 469-475.
[199] Dolcetti R, Viel A, Doglioni C et al. High prevalence of activated intraepithelial cytotoxic T lymphocytes and increased neoplastic cell apoptosis in colorectal carcinomas with microsatellite instability. *Am. J. Pathol.* 1999; 154: 1805-1813.
[200] Velayos FS, Lee SH, Qiu H et al. The Mechanism of Microsatellite Instability Is Different in Synchronous and Metachronous *Colorectal Cancer. J. Gastrointest. Surg.* 2005; 9: 329-335.
[201] Haddad R, Ogilvie RT, Croitoru M et al. Microsatellite instability as a prognostic factor in resected colorectal cancer liver metastases. *Ann. Surg. Oncol.* 2004; 11:977-982.

[202] Bacher JW, Flanagan LA, Smalley RL et al. Development of a fluorescent multiplex assay for detection of MSI-High tumors. *Dis. Markers.* 2004; 20: 237-250.

[203] Buhard O, Suraweera N, Lectard A et al. Quasimonomorphic mononucleotide repeats for high-level microsatellite instability analysis. *Dis. Markers.* 2004; 20: 251-257.

[204] Gologan A, Sepulveda AR. Microsatellite instability and DNA mismatch repair deficiency testing in hereditary and sporadic gastrointestinal cancers. *Clin. Lab. Med.* 2005; 25: 179-196.

[205] Hatch SB, Lightfoot HM, Jr., Garwacki CP et al. Microsatellite instability testing in colorectal carcinoma: choice of markers affects sensitivity of detection of mismatch repair-deficient tumors. *Clin. Cancer Res.* 2005; 11: 2180-2187.

[206] Rodriguez-Bigas MA, Boland CR, Hamilton SR et al. A National Cancer Institute Workshop on Hereditary Nonpolyposis Colorectal Cancer Syndrome: meeting highlights and Bethesda guidelines. *J. Natl. Cancer Inst.* 1997; 89: 1758-1762.

[207] Chapusot C, Martin L, Puig PL et al. What is the best way to assess microsatellite instability status in colorectal cancer? Study on a population base of 462 colorectal cancers. *Am. J. Surg. Pathol.* 2004; 28: 1553-1559.

[208] Chaves P, Cruz C, Lage P et al. Immunohistochemical detection of mismatch repair gene proteins as a useful tool for the identification of colorectal carcinoma with the mutator phenotype. *J. Pathol.* 2000; 191: 355-360.

[209] Liu T, Wahlberg S, Burek E et al. Microsatellite instability as a predictor of a mutation in a DNA mismatch repair gene in familial colorectal cancer. *Genes Chromosomes Cancer.* 2000; 27: 17-25.

[210] Shia J, Ellis NA, Paty PB et al. Value of histopathology in predicting microsatellite instability in hereditary nonpolyposis colorectal cancer and sporadic colorectal cancer. *Am. J. Surg. Pathol.* 2003; 27: 1407-1417.

[211] Nash GM, Gimbel M, Shia J et al. Automated, multiplex assay for high-frequency microsatellite instability in colorectal cancer. *J. Clin. Oncol.* 2003; 21: 3105-3112.

[212] Umetani N, Sasaki S, Watanabe T et al. Diagnostic primer sets for microsatellite instability optimized for a minimal amount of damaged DNA from colorectal tissue samples. *Ann. Surg. Oncol.* 2000; 7: 276-280.

[213] Halford SE, Sawyer EJ, Lambros MB et al. MSI-low, a real phenomenon which varies in frequency among cancer types. *J. Pathol.* 2003; 201: 389-394.

[214] Jass JR, Young J, Leggett BA. Biological significance of microsatellite instability-low (MSI-L) status in colorectal tumors. *Am. J. Pathol.* 2001; 158: 779-781.
[215] Pawlik TM, Raut CP, Rodriguez-Bigas MA. Colorectal carcinogenesis: MSI-H versus MSI-L. *Dis. Markers.* 2004; 20: 199-206.
[216] Halford S, Sasieni P, Rowan A et al. Low-level microsatellite instability occurs in most colorectal cancers and is a nonrandomly distributed quantitative trait. *Cancer Res.* 2002; 62: 53-57.
[217] Oda S, Maehara Y, Ikeda Y et al. Two modes of microsatellite instability in human cancer: differential connection of defective DNA mismatch repair to dinucleotide repeat instability. *Nucleic Acids Res.* 2005; 33: 1628-1636.
[218] Oda S, Maehara Y, Sumiyoshi Y, Sugimachi K. Microsatellite instability in cancer: what problems remain unanswered? *Surgery.* 2002; 131: S55-62.
[219] Suraweera N, Duval A, Reperant M et al. Evaluation of tumor microsatellite instability using five quasimonomorphic mononucleotide repeats and pentaplex PCR. *Gastroenterology.* 2002; 123: 1804-1811.
[220] Whitehall VL, Walsh MD, Young J et al. Methylation of O-6-methylguanine DNA methyltransferase characterizes a subset of colorectal cancer with low-level DNA microsatellite instability. *Cancer Res.* 2001; 61: 827-830.
[221] Kimura N, Nagasaka T, Murakami J et al. Methylation profiles of genes utilizing newly developed CpG island methylation microarray on colorectal cancer patients. *Nucleic Acids Res.* 2005; 33: e46.
[222] Feinberg AP, Ohlsson R, Henikoff S. The epigenetic progenitor origin of human cancer. *Nat. Rev. Genet.* 2006; 7: 21-33.
[223] Epigenetic markers in the detection of colorectal cancer. *Nat. Clin. Pract. Gastroenterol. Hepatol.* 2005; 2: 126.
[224] Grady WM. Epigenetic events in the colorectum and in colon cancer. *Biochem. Soc. Trans.* 2005; 33: 684-688.
[225] Clarke MF. Epigenetic regulation of normal and cancer stem cells. *Ann. N. Y. Acad. Sci.* 2005; 1044: 90-93.
[226] Frigola J, Song J, Stirzaker C et al. Epigenetic remodeling in colorectal cancer results in coordinate gene suppression across an entire chromosome band. *Nat. Genet.* 2006; 38: 540-549.
[227] Baylin SB, Ohm JE. Epigenetic gene silencing in cancer - a mechanism for early oncogenic pathway addiction? *Nat. Rev. Cancer.* 2006; 6: 107-116.

[228] Tomasi TB, Magner WJ, Khan AN. Epigenetic regulation of immune escape genes in cancer. *Cancer Immunol. Immunother.* 2006.

[229] Lyko F, Brown R. DNA methyltransferase inhibitors and the development of epigenetic cancer therapies. *J. Natl. Cancer Inst.* 2005; 97: 1498-1506.

[230] Sigalotti L, Coral S, Fratta E et al. Epigenetic modulation of solid tumors as a novel approach for cancer immunotherapy. *Semin. Oncol.* 2005; 32: 473-478.

[231] Miyakura Y, Sugano K, Akasu T et al. Extensive but hemiallelic methylation of the hMLH1 promoter region in early-onset sporadic colon cancers with microsatellite instability. *Clin. Gastroenterol. Hepatol.* 2004; 2: 147-156.

[232] Herman JG, Baylin SB. Gene silencing in cancer in association with promoter hypermethylation. *N. Engl. J. Med.* 2003; 349: 2042-2054.

[233] Herman JG, Umar A, Polyak K et al. Incidence and functional consequences of hMLH1 promoter hypermethylation in colorectal carcinoma. *Proc. Natl. Acad. Sci. U. S. A.* 1998; 95: 6870-6875.

[234] Wheeler JM, Loukola A, Aaltonen LA et al. The role of hypermethylation of the hMLH1 promoter region in HNPCC versus MSI+ sporadic colorectal cancers. *J. Med. Genet.* 2000; 37: 588-592.

[235] Kondo Y, Issa JP. Epigenetic changes in colorectal cancer. *Cancer Metastasis Rev.* 2004; 23: 29-39.

[236] Toyota M, Ahuja N, Ohe-Toyota M et al. CpG island methylator phenotype in colorectal cancer. *Proc. Natl. Acad. Sci. U. S. A.* 1999; 96: 8681-8686.

[237] Lin SY, Yeh KT, Chen WT et al. Promoter CpG methylation of tumor suppressor genes in colorectal cancer and its relationship to clinical features. *Oncol. Rep.* 2004; 11: 341-348.

[238] Lind GE, Thorstensen L, Lovig T et al. A CpG island hypermethylation profile of primary colorectal carcinomas and colon cancer cell lines. *Mol. Cancer.* 2004; 3: 28.

[239] Van Rijnsoever M, Elsaleh H, Joseph D et al. CpG island methylator phenotype is an independent predictor of survival benefit from 5-fluorouracil in stage III colorectal cancer. *Clin. Cancer Res.* 2003; 9: 2898-2903.

[240] Kuismanen SA, Holmberg MT, Salovaara R et al. Genetic and epigenetic modification of MLH1 accounts for a major share of microsatellite-unstable colorectal cancers. *Am. J. Pathol.* 2000; 156: 1773-1779.

[241] Ward RL, Cheong K, Ku SL et al. Adverse prognostic effect of methylation in colorectal cancer is reversed by microsatellite instability. *J. Clin. Oncol.* 2003; 21: 3729-3736.

[242] Jass JR. Serrated adenoma of the colorectum and the DNA-methylator phenotype. *Nat. Clin. Pract. Oncol.* 2005; 2: 398-405.

[243] Oh K, Redston M, Odze RD. Support for hMLH1 and MGMT silencing as a mechanism of tumorigenesis in the hyperplastic-adenoma-carcinoma (serrated) carcinogenic pathway in the colon. *Hum. Pathol.* 2005; 36: 101-111.

[244] Lazarus R, Junttila OE, Karttunen TJ, Makinen MJ. The risk of metachronous neoplasia in patients with serrated adenoma. *Am. J. Clin. Pathol* 2005; 123: 349-359.

[245] Jass JR. Serrated adenoma of the colorectum: a lesion with teeth. *Am J Pathol.* 2003; 162: 705-708.

[246] Horkko TT, Makinen MJ. Colorectal proliferation and apoptosis in serrated versus conventional adenoma-carcinoma pathway: growth, progression and survival. *Scand. J. Gastroenterol.* 2003; 38: 1241-1248.

[247] Tateyama H, Li W, Takahashi E et al. Apoptosis index and apoptosis-related antigen expression in serrated adenoma of the colorectum: the saw-toothed structure may be related to inhibition of apoptosis. *Am. J. Surg. Pathol.* 2002; 26: 249-256.

[248] Oka S, Tanaka S, Hiyama T et al. Human telomerase reverse transcriptase, p53 and Ki-67 expression and apoptosis in colorectal serrated adenoma. *Scand. J. Gastroenterol.* 2002; 37: 1194-1200.

[249] Morita T, Tamura S, Miyazaki J et al. Evaluation of endoscopic and histopathological features of serrated adenoma of the colon. *Endoscopy.* 2001; 33: 761-765.

[250] Makinen MJ, George SM, Jernvall P et al. Colorectal carcinoma associated with serrated adenoma--prevalence, histological features, and prognosis. *J. Pathol.* 2001; 193: 286-294.

[251] Arao J, Sano Y, Fujii T et al. Cyclooxygenase-2 is overexpressed in serrated adenoma of the colorectum. *Dis. Colon. Rectum.* 2001; 44: 1319-1323.

[252] Jass JR. Serrated adenoma and colorectal cancer. *J. Pathol.* 1999; 187: 499-502.

[253] Snover DC, Jass JR, Fenoglio-Preiser C, Batts KP. Serrated polyps of the large intestine: a morphologic and molecular review of an evolving concept. *Am. J. Clin. Pathol.* 2005; 124: 380-391.

[254] Longacre TA, Fenoglio-Preiser CM. Mixed hyperplastic adenomatous polyps/serrated adenomas. A distinct form of colorectal neoplasia. *Am. J. Surg. Pathol.* 1990; 14:524-537.

[255] Fenoglio-Preiser CM. When is a hyperplastic polyp not a hyperplastic polyp? *Am. J. Surg. Pathol.* 1999; 23: 1001-1003.

[256] Park SY, Lee HS, Choe G et al. Clinicopathological characteristics, microsatellite instability, and expression of mucin core proteins and p53 in colorectal mucinous adenocarcinomas in relation to location. *Virchows Arch.* 2006.

[257] Tatsumi N, Mukaisho K, Mitsufuji S et al. Expression of cytokeratins 7 and 20 in serrated adenoma and related diseases. *Dig. Dis. Sci.* 2005; 50: 1741-1746.

[258] Hohenstein P, Molenaar L, Elsinga J et al. Serrated adenomas and mixed polyposis caused by a splice acceptor deletion in the mouse Smad4 gene. *Genes Chromosomes Cancer.* 2003; 36: 273-282.

[259] Thun MJ, Namboodiri MM, Heath CW, Jr. Aspirin use and reduced risk of fatal colon cancer. *N. Engl. J. Med.* 1991; 325: 1593-1596.

[260] Phillips RK, Wallace MH, Lynch PM et al. A randomised, double blind, placebo controlled study of celecoxib, a selective cyclooxygenase 2 inhibitor, on duodenal polyposis in familial adenomatous polyposis. *Gut.* 2002; 50: 857-860.

[261] Thun MJ, Henley SJ, Patrono C. Nonsteroidal anti-inflammatory drugs as anticancer agents: mechanistic, pharmacologic, and clinical issues. *J. Natl. Cancer Inst.* 2002; 94: 252-266.

[262] Baron JA, Cole BF, Sandler RS et al. A randomized trial of aspirin to prevent colorectal adenomas. *N. Engl. J. Med.* 2003; 348: 891-899.

[263] Bresalier RS SR, Bolognese J, et al. A randmized trial of rofecoxib to prevent colorectal adenomas. *Gastroenterology.* 2005; 128: A 35.

[264] Reddy BS. Studies with the azoxymethane-rat preclinical model for assessing colon tumor development and chemoprevention. *Environ. Mol. Mutagen.* 2004; 44: 26-35.

[265] Yao M, Kargman S, Lam EC et al. Inhibition of cyclooxygenase-2 by rofecoxib attenuates the growth and metastatic potential of colorectal carcinoma in mice. *Cancer Res.* 2003; 63: 586-592.

[266] Sonoshita M, Takaku K, Sasaki N et al. Acceleration of intestinal polyposis through prostaglandin receptor EP2 in Apc(Delta 716) knockout mice. *Nat. Med.* 2001; 7: 1048-1051.

[267] Mutoh M, Watanabe K, Kitamura T et al. Involvement of prostaglandin E receptor subtype EP(4) in colon carcinogenesis. *Cancer Res.* 2002; 62: 28-32.

[268] Charalambous MP, Maihofner C, Bhambra U et al. Upregulation of cyclooxygenase-2 is accompanied by increased expression of nuclear factor-kappa B and I kappa B kinase-alpha in human colorectal cancer epithelial cells. *Br. J. Cancer.* 2003; 88: 1598-1604.

[269] Sheng H, Shao J, Kirkland SC et al. Inhibition of human colon cancer cell growth by selective inhibition of cyclooxygenase-2. *J. Clin. Invest.* 1997; 99: 2254-2259.

[270] Konturek PC, Kania J, Burnat G et al. Prostaglandins as mediators of COX-2 derived *carcinogenesis* in gastrointestinal tract. *J. Physiol. Pharmacol.* 2005; 56 Suppl 5: 57-73.

[271] Gupta RA, Dubois RN. Colorectal cancer prevention and treatment by inhibition of cyclooxygenase-2. *Nat. Rev. Cancer.* 2001; 1: 11-21.

[272] Harris RE, Alshafie GA, Abou-Issa H, Seibert K. Chemoprevention of breast cancer in rats by celecoxib, a cyclooxygenase 2 inhibitor. *Cancer Res.* 2000; 60: 2101-2103.

[273] Oshima M, Murai N, Kargman S et al. Chemoprevention of intestinal polyposis in the Apcdelta716 mouse by rofecoxib, a specific cyclooxygenase-2 inhibitor. *Cancer Res.* 2001; 61: 1733-1740.

[274] Eisinger AL, Nadauld LD, Shelton DN et al. The APC tumor suppressor gene regulates expression of cyclooxygenase-2 by a mechanism that involves retinoic acid. *J. Biol. Chem.* 2006.

[275] Oshima M, Dinchuk JE, Kargman SL et al. Suppression of intestinal polyposis in Apc delta716 knockout mice by inhibition of cyclooxygenase 2 (COX-2). *Cell.* 1996; 87: 803-809.

[276] Jacoby RF, Cole CE, Tutsch K et al. Chemopreventive efficacy of combined piroxicam and difluoromethylornithine treatment of Apc mutant Min mouse adenomas, and selective toxicity against Apc mutant embryos. *Cancer Res.* 2000; 60: 1864-1870.

[277] Jacoby RF, Seibert K, Cole CE et al. The cyclooxygenase-2 inhibitor celecoxib is a potent preventive and therapeutic agent in the min mouse model of adenomatous polyposis. *Cancer Res.* 2000; 60: 5040-5044.

[278] Kawamori T, Rao CV, Seibert K, Reddy BS. Chemopreventive activity of celecoxib, a specific cyclooxygenase-2 inhibitor, against colon carcinogenesis. *Cancer Res.* 1998; 58: 409-412.

[279] Araki Y, Okamura S, Hussain SP et al. Regulation of cyclooxygenase-2 expression by the Wnt and ras pathways. *Cancer Res.* 2003; 63: 728-734.

[280] Dubois RN, Abramson SB, Crofford L et al. Cyclooxygenase in biology and disease. *Faseb. J.* 1998; 12: 1063-1073.
[281] Tanabe T, Tohnai N. Cyclooxygenase isozymes and their gene structures and expression. Prostaglandins *Other Lipid Mediat.* 2002; 68-69: 95-114.
[282] Xu XL, Yu J, Zhang HY et al. Methylation profile of the promoter CpG islands of 31 genes that may contribute to colorectal carcinogenesis. *World J. Gastroenterol.* 2004; 10: 3441-3454.
[283] Dixon DA, Kaplan CD, McIntyre TM et al. Post-transcriptional control of cyclooxygenase-2 gene expression. The role of the 3'-untranslated region. *J. Biol. Chem.* 2000; 275: 11750-11757.
[284] Dixon DA, Tolley ND, King PH et al. Altered expression of the mRNA stability factor HuR promotes cyclooxygenase-2 expression in colon cancer cells. *J. Clin. Invest.* 2001; 108: 1657-1665.
[285] Sheng H, Shao J, Dubois RN. K-Ras-mediated increase in cyclooxygenase 2 mRNA stability involves activation of the protein kinase B1. *Cancer Res.* 2001; 61: 2670-2675.
[286] Dixon DA, Balch GC, Kedersha N et al. Regulation of cyclooxygenase-2 expression by the translational silencer TIA-1. *J. Exp. Med.* 2003; 198: 475-481.
[287] Wang D, Mann JR, DuBois RN. The role of prostaglandins and other eicosanoids in the gastrointestinal tract. *Gastroenterology.* 2005; 128: 1445-1461.
[288] Levy GN. Prostaglandin H synthases, nonsteroidal anti-inflammatory drugs, and colon cancer. *Faseb. J.* 1997; 11: 234-247.
[289] Smith WL, DeWitt DL, Garavito RM. Cyclooxygenases: structural, cellular, and molecular biology. *Annu. Rev. Biochem.* 2000; 69: 145-182.
[290] Williams CS, DuBois RN. Prostaglandin endoperoxide synthase: why two isoforms? *Am. J. Physiol.* 1996; 270: G393-400.
[291] Subbaramaiah K, Telang N, Ramonetti JT et al. Transcription of cyclooxygenase-2 is enhanced in transformed mammary epithelial cells. *Cancer Res.* 1996; 56: 4424-4429.
[292] Eberhart CE, Coffey RJ, Radhika A et al. Up-regulation of cyclooxygenase 2 gene expression in human colorectal adenomas and adenocarcinomas. *Gastroenterology.* 1994; 107: 1183-1188.
[293] Sinicrope FA, Lemoine M, Xi L et al. Reduced expression of cyclooxygenase 2 proteins in hereditary nonpolyposis colorectal cancers relative to sporadic cancers. *Gastroenterology.* 1999; 117: 350-358.

[294] Singer, II, Kawka DW, Schloemann S et al. Cyclooxygenase 2 is induced in colonic epithelial cells in inflammatory bowel disease. *Gastroenterology.* 1998; 115: 297-306.

[295] Pugh S, Thomas GA. Patients with adenomatous polyps and carcinomas have increased colonic mucosal prostaglandin E2. *Gut.* 1994; 35: 675-678.

[296] Rigas B, Goldman IS, Levine L. Altered eicosanoid levels in human colon cancer. *J. Lab. Clin. Med.* 1993; 122: 518-523.

[297] Chi Y, Khersonsky SM, Chang YT, Schuster VL. Identification of a new class of prostaglandin transporter inhibitors and characterization of their biological effects on prostaglandin E2 transport. *J. Pharmacol. Exp. Ther.* 2006; 316: 1346-1350.

[298] Kudo I, Murakami M. Phospholipase A2 enzymes. *Prostaglandins Other Lipid Mediat.* 2002; 68-69: 3-58.

[299] Sinicrope FA, Gill S. Role of cyclooxygenase-2 in colorectal cancer. *Cancer Metastasis Rev.* 2004; 23: 63-75.

[300] Breyer RM, Bagdassarian CK, Myers SA, Breyer MD. Prostanoid receptors: subtypes and signaling. *Annu. Rev. Pharmacol. Toxicol.* 2001; 41: 661-690.

[301] Tetsu O, McCormick F. Beta-catenin regulates expression of cyclin D1 in colon carcinoma cells. *Nature.* 1999; 398: 422-426.

[302] Castellone MD, Teramoto H, Williams BO et al. Prostaglandin E2 promotes colon cancer cell growth through a Gs-axin-beta-catenin signaling axis. *Science.* 2005; 310: 1504-1510.

[303] Mei JM, Hord NG, Winterstein DF et al. Differential expression of prostaglandin endoperoxide H synthase-2 and formation of activated beta-catenin-LEF-1 transcription complex in mouse colonic epithelial cells contrasting in Apc. *Carcinogenesis.* 1999; 20: 737-740.

[304] Fujino H, Srinivasan D, Regan JW. Cellular conditioning and activation of beta-catenin signaling by the FPB prostanoid receptor. *J. Biol. Chem.* 2002; 277: 48786-48795.

[305] Fujino H, West KA, Regan JW. Phosphorylation of glycogen synthase kinase-3 and stimulation of T-cell factor signaling following activation of EP2 and EP4 prostanoid receptors by prostaglandin E2. *J. Biol. Chem.* 2002; 277: 2614-2619.

[306] Pai R, Soreghan B, Szabo IL et al. Prostaglandin E2 transactivates EGF receptor: a novel mechanism for promoting colon cancer growth and gastrointestinal hypertrophy. *Nat. Med.* 2002; 8: 289-293.

[307] Dannenberg AJ, Lippman SM, Mann JR et al. Cyclooxygenase-2 and epidermal growth factor receptor: pharmacologic targets for chemoprevention. *J. Clin. Oncol.* 2005; 23: 254-266.
[308] Ceccarelli C, Piazzi G, Paterini P et al. Concurrent EGFr and Cox-2 expression in colorectal cancer: proliferation impact and tumour spreading. *Ann. Oncol.* 2005; 16 Suppl 4: iv74-iv79.
[309] Shao J, Lee SB, Guo H et al. Prostaglandin E2 stimulates the growth of colon cancer cells via induction of amphiregulin. *Cancer Res.* 2003; 63: 5218-5223.
[310] Buchanan FG, DuBois RN. Connecting COX-2 and Wnt in cancer. *Cancer. Cell* 2006; 9: 6-8.
[311] Sun Y, Tang XM, Half E et al. Cyclooxygenase-2 overexpression reduces apoptotic susceptibility by inhibiting the cytochrome c-dependent apoptotic pathway in human colon cancer cells. *Cancer Res.* 2002; 62: 6323-6328.
[312] Tang X, Sun YJ, Half E et al. Cyclooxygenase-2 overexpression inhibits death receptor 5 expression and confers resistance to tumor necrosis factor-related apoptosis-inducing ligand-induced apoptosis in human colon cancer cells. *Cancer Res.* 2002; 62: 4903-4908.
[313] Sheng H, Shao J, Morrow JD et al. Modulation of apoptosis and Bcl-2 expression by prostaglandin E2 in human colon cancer cells. *Cancer Res.* 1998; 58: 362-366.
[314] Tsujii M, DuBois RN. Alterations in cellular adhesion and apoptosis in epithelial cells overexpressing prostaglandin endoperoxide synthase 2. *Cell.* 1995; 83: 493-501.
[315] Nzeako UC, Guicciardi ME, Yoon JH et al. COX-2 inhibits Fas-mediated apoptosis in cholangiocarcinoma cells. *Hepatology.* 2002; 35: 552-559.
[316] McGill G, Fisher DE. Apoptosis in tumorigenesis and cancer therapy. *Front Biosci.* 1997; 2: d353-379.
[317] Beltrami E, Plescia J, Wilkinson JC et al. Acute ablation of survivin uncovers p53-dependent mitotic checkpoint functions and control of mitochondrial apoptosis. *J. Biol. Chem.* 2004; 279: 2077-2084.
[318] Benoit V, de Moraes E, Dar NA et al. Transcriptional activation of cyclooxygenase-2 by tumor suppressor p53 requires nuclear factor-kappaB. *Oncogene.* 2006.
[319] Chang SH, Liu CH, Conway R et al. Role of prostaglandin E2-dependent angiogenic switch in cyclooxygenase 2-induced breast cancer progression. *Proc. Natl. Acad. Sci. U. S. A.* 2004; 101: 591-596.

[320] Wang D, DuBois RN. Cyclooxygenase 2-derived prostaglandin E2 regulates the angiogenic switch. *Proc. Natl. Acad. Sci. U. S. A.* 2004; 101: 415-416.

[321] DeClerck YA, Mercurio AM, Stack MS et al. Proteases, extracellular matrix, and cancer: a workshop of the path B study section. *Am. J. Pathol.* 2004; 164: 1131-1139.

[322] Borg TK. It's the matrix! ECM, proteases, and cancer. *Am. J. Pathol.* 2004; 164: 1141-1142.

[323] Itkonen O, Stenman UH, Osman S et al. Serum samples from pancreatectomized patients contain trypsinogen immunoreactivity. *J. Lab. Clin. Med.* 1996; 128: 98-102.

[324] Koshikawa N, Hasegawa S, Nagashima Y et al. Expression of trypsin by epithelial cells of various tissues, leukocytes, and neurons in human and mouse. *Am. J. Pathol.* 1998; 153: 937-944.

[325] Emi M, Nakamura Y, Ogawa M et al. Cloning, characterization and nucleotide sequences of two cDNAs encoding human pancreatic trypsinogens. *Gene.* 1986; 41: 305-310.

[326] Tani T, Kawashima I, Mita K, Takiguchi Y. Nucleotide sequence of the human pancreatic trypsinogen III cDNA. *Nucleic Acids Res.* 1990; 18: 1631.

[327] Wiegand U, Corbach S, Minn A et al. Cloning of the cDNA encoding human brain trypsinogen and characterization of its product. *Gene.* 1993; 136: 167-175.

[328] Imamura T, Kitamoto Y. Expression of enteropeptidase in differentiated enterocytes, goblet cells, and the tumor cells in human duodenum. *Am. J. Physiol. Gastrointest. Liver Physiol.* 2003; 285: G1235-1241.

[329] Miyata S, Koshikawa N, Higashi S et al. Expression of trypsin in human cancer cell lines and cancer tissues and its tight binding to soluble form of Alzheimer amyloid precursor protein in culture. *J. Biochem. (Tokyo)* 1999; 125: 1067-1076.

[330] O'Keefe S J, Lee RB, Li J et al. Trypsin Secretion and Turnover in Patients with Acute Pancreatitis. *Am. J. Physiol. Gastrointest. Liver Physiol.* 2005.

[331] Descamps FJ, Martens E, Ballaux F et al. In vivo activation of gelatinase B/MMP-9 by trypsin in acute pancreatitis is a permissive factor in streptozotocin-induced diabetes. *J. Pathol.* 2004; 204: 555-561.

[332] Howes N, Greenhalf W, Stocken DD, Neoptolemos JP. Cationic trypsinogen mutations and pancreatitis. *Gastroenterol. Clin. North Am.* 2004; 33: 767-787.

[333] Stenman UH, Koivunen E, Itkonen O. Biology and function of tumor-associated trypsin inhibitor, TATI. *Scand. J. Clin. Lab. Invest. Suppl.* 1991; 207: 5-9.

[334] Hirahara F, Miyagi E, Nagashima Y et al. Differential expression of trypsin in human ovarian carcinomas and low-malignant-potential tumors. *Gynecol. Oncol.* 1998; 68: 162-165.

[335] Paju A, Vartiainen J, Haglund C et al. Expression of trypsinogen-1, trypsinogen-2, and tumor-associated trypsin inhibitor in ovarian cancer: prognostic study on tissue and serum. *Clin. Cancer Res.* 2004; 10: 4761-4768.

[336] Bjartell A, Paju A, Zhang WM et al. Expression of tumor-associated trypsinogens (TAT-1 and TAT-2) in prostate cancer. *Prostate.* 2005.

[337] Kawano N, Osawa H, Ito T et al. Expression of gelatinase A, tissue inhibitor of metalloproteinases-2, matrilysin, and trypsin(ogen) in lung neoplasms: an immunohistochemical study. *Hum. Pathol.* 1997; 28: 613-622.

[338] Kato Y, Nagashima Y, Koshikawa N et al. Production of trypsins by human gastric cancer cells correlates with their malignant phenotype. *Eur. J. Cancer.* 1998; 34: 1117-1123.

[339] Koivunen E, Saksela O, Itkonen O et al. Human colon carcinoma, fibrosarcoma and leukemia cell lines produce tumor-associated trypsinogen. *Int. J. Cancer.* 1991; 47: 592-596.

[340] Yamamoto H, Iku S, Adachi Y et al. Association of trypsin expression with tumour progression and matrilysin expression in human colorectal cancer. *J. Pathol.* 2003; 199: 176-184.

[341] Koivunen E, Ristimaki A, Itkonen O et al. Tumor-associated trypsin participates in cancer cell-mediated degradation of extracellular matrix. *Cancer Res.* 1991; 51: 2107-2112.

[342] Sorsa T, Salo T, Koivunen E et al. Activation of type IV procollagenases by human tumor-associated trypsin-2. *J. Biol. Chem.* 1997; 272: 21067-21074.

[343] Alm AK, Gagnemo-Persson R, Sorsa T, Sundelin J. Extrapancreatic trypsin-2 cleaves proteinase-activated receptor-2. *Biochem. Biophys. Res. Commun.* 2000; 275: 77-83.

[344] Lukkonen A, Sorsa T, Salo T et al. Down-regulation of trypsinogen-2 expression by chemically modified tetracyclines: association with reduced cancer cell migration. *Int. J. Cancer.* 2000; 86: 577-581.

[345] Moilanen M, Sorsa T, Stenman M et al. Tumor-associated trypsinogen-2 (trypsinogen-2) activates procollagenases (MMP-1, -8, -13) and stromelysin-1 (MMP-3) and degrades type I collagen. *Biochemistry.* 2003; 42: 5414-5420.

[346] Verspaget HW. Proteases as prognostic markers in cancer. *BMJ.* 1998; 316: 790-791.

[347] Heslin MJ, Yan J, Johnson MR et al. Role of matrix metalloproteinases in colorectal carcinogenesis. *Ann. Surg.* 2001; 233: 786-792.

[348] Mueller MM, Fusenig NE. Friends or foes - bipolar effects of the tumour stroma in cancer. *Nat. Rev. Cancer.* 2004; 4: 839-849.

[349] Boedefeld WM, 2nd, Bland KI, Heslin MJ. Recent insights into angiogenesis, apoptosis, invasion, and metastasis in colorectal carcinoma. *Ann. Surg. Oncol.* 2003; 10: 839-851.

[350] Leeman MF, Curran S, Murray GI. New insights into the roles of matrix metalloproteinases in colorectal cancer development and progression. *J. Pathol.* 2003; 201: 528-534.

[351] Moran A, Iniesta P, Garcia-Aranda C et al. Clinical relevance of MMP-9, MMP-2, TIMP-1 and TIMP-2 in colorectal cancer. *Oncol. Rep.* 2005; 13: 115-120.

[352] Kioi M, Yamamoto K, Higashi S et al. Matrilysin (MMP-7) induces homotypic adhesion of human colon cancer cells and enhances their metastatic potential in nude mouse model. *Oncogene* 2003; 22: 8662-8670.

[353] Turpeinen U, Koivunen E, Stenman UH. Reaction of a tumour-associated trypsin inhibitor with serine proteinases associated with coagulation and tumour invasion. *Biochem. J.* 1988; 254: 911-914.

[354] Nyberg P, Moilanen M, Paju A et al. MMP-9 activation by tumor trypsin-2 enhances in vivo invasion of human tongue carcinoma cells. *J. Dent. Res.* 2002; 81: 831-835.

[355] Nishibori M, Mori S, Takahashi HK. Physiology and pathophysiology of proteinase-activated receptors (PARs): PAR-2-mediated proliferation of colon cancer cell. *J. Pharmacol. Sci.* 2005; 97: 25-30.

[356] Yada K, Shibata K, Matsumoto T et al. Protease-activated receptor-2 regulates cell proliferation and enhances cyclooxygenase-2 mRNA expression in human pancreatic cancer cells. *J. Surg. Oncol.* 2005; 89: 79-85.

[357] Darmoul D, Gratio V, Devaud H, Laburthe M. Protease-activated receptor 2 in colon cancer: trypsin-induced MAPK phosphorylation and cell proliferation are mediated by epidermal growth factor receptor transactivation. *J. Biol. Chem.* 2004; 279: 20927-20934.

[358] Williams SJ, Gotley DC, Antalis TM. Human trypsinogen in colorectal cancer. *Int. J. Cancer.* 2001; 93: 67-73.

[359] Solakidi S, Tiniakos DG, Petraki K et al. Co-expression of trypsin and tumour-associated trypsin inhibitor (TATI) in colorectal adenocarcinomas. *Histol. Histopathol.* 2003; 18: 1181-1188.

[360] Yamashita K, Mimori K, Inoue H et al. A tumor-suppressive role for trypsin in human cancer progression. *Cancer Res.* 2003; 63: 6575-6578.

[361] Uchima Y, Sawada T, Nishihara T et al. Identification of a trypsinogen activity stimulating factor produced by pancreatic cancer cells: its role in tumor invasion and metastasis. *Int. J. Mol. Med.* 2003; 12: 871-878.

[362] Ducroc R, Bontemps C, Marazova K et al. Trypsin is produced by and activates protease-activated receptor-2 in human cancer colon cells: evidence for new autocrine loop. *Life Sci.* 2002; 70: 1359-1367.

[363] Bohe H, Bohe M, Lindstrom C, Ohlsson K. Immunohistochemical demonstration of pancreatic secretory trypsin inhibitor in normal and neoplastic colonic mucosa. *J. Clin. Pathol.* 1990; 43: 901-904.

[364] Bohe M, Borgstrom A, Lindstrom C, Ohlsson K. Pancreatic endoproteases and pancreatic secretory trypsin inhibitor immunoreactivity in human Paneth cells. *J. Clin. Pathol.* 1986; 39: 786-793.

[365] Tomita N, Doi S, Higashiyama M et al. Expression of pancreatic secretory trypsin inhibitor gene in human colorectal tumor. *Cancer.* 1990; 66: 2144-2149.

[366] Higashiyama M, Monden T, Tomita N et al. Expression of pancreatic secretory trypsin inhibitor (PSTI) in colorectal cancer. *Br. J. Cancer.* 1990; 62: 954-958.

[367] Solakidi S, Dessypris A, Stathopoulos GP et al. Tumour-associated trypsin inhibitor, carcinoembryonic antigen and acute-phase reactant proteins CRP and alpha1-antitrypsin in patients with gastrointestinal malignancies. *Clin. Biochem.* 2004; 37:56-60.

[368] Zucker S, Vacirca J. Role of matrix metalloproteinases (MMPs) in colorectal cancer. *Cancer Metastasis. Rev.* 2004; 23: 101-117.

[369] Wagenaar-Miller RA, Gordon L, Matrisian LM. Matrix metalloproteinases in colorectal cancer: Is it worth talking about? *Cancer Metastasis Rev.* 2004; 23: 119-135.

[370] Coussens LM, Fingleton B, Matrisian LM. Matrix metalloproteinase inhibitors and cancer: trials and tribulations. *Science.* 2002; 295: 2387-2392.

[371] Zinzindohoue F, Lecomte T, Ferraz JM et al. Prognostic significance of MMP-1 and MMP-3 functional promoter polymorphisms in colorectal cancer. *Clin. Cancer Res.* 2005; 11: 594-599.

[372] Zeng ZS, Shu WP, Cohen AM, Guillem JG. Matrix metalloproteinase-7 expression in colorectal cancer liver metastases: evidence for involvement of MMP-7 activation in human cancer metastases. *Clin Cancer Res.* 2002; 8: 144-148.

[373] Zeng ZS, Huang Y, Cohen AM, Guillem JG. Prediction of colorectal cancer relapse and survival via tissue RNA levels of matrix metalloproteinase-9. *J. Clin. Oncol.* 1996; 14: 3133-3140.

[374] Witty JP, McDonnell S, Newell KJ et al. Modulation of matrilysin levels in colon carcinoma cell lines affects tumorigenicity in vivo. *Cancer Res.* 1994; 54: 4805-4812.

[375] Tien YW, Lee PH, Hu RH et al. The role of gelatinase in hepatic metastasis of colorectal cancer. *Clin. Cancer Res.* 2003; 9: 4891-4896.

[376] Matsuyama Y, Takao S, Aikou T. Comparison of matrix metalloproteinase expression between primary tumors with or without liver metastasis in pancreatic and colorectal carcinomas. *J. Surg. Oncol.* 2002; 80: 105-110.

[377] Masaki T, Sugiyama M, Matsuoka H et al. Coexpression of matrilysin and laminin-5 gamma2 chain may contribute to tumor cell migration in colorectal carcinomas. *Dig. Dis. Sci.* 2003; 48: 1262-1267.

[378] Masaki T, Sugiyama M, Matsuoka H et al. Matrix metalloproteinases may contribute compensationally to tumor invasion in T1 colorectal carcinomas. *Anticancer Res.* 2003; 23: 4169-4173.

[379] Masaki T, Matsuoka H, Sugiyama M et al. Laminin-5 gamma 2 chain and matrix metalloproteinase-2 may trigger colorectal carcinoma invasiveness through formation of budding tumor cells. *Anticancer Res.* 2003; 23: 4113-4119.

[380] Masaki T, Matsuoka H, Sugiyama M et al. Matrilysin (MMP-7) as a significant determinant of malignant potential of early invasive colorectal carcinomas. *Br. J. Cancer.* 2001; 84: 1317-1321.

[381] Leeman MF, McKay JA, Murray GI. Matrix metalloproteinase 13 activity is associated with poor prognosis in colorectal cancer. *J. Clin. Pathol.* 2002; 55: 758-762.

[382] Itoh F, Yamamoto H, Hinoda Y, Imai K. Enhanced secretion and activation of matrilysin during malignant conversion of human colorectal epithelium and its relationship with invasive potential of colon cancer cells. *Cancer.* 1996; 77: 1717-1721.

[383] Imai K, Yokohama Y, Nakanishi I et al. Matrix metalloproteinase 7 (matrilysin) from human rectal carcinoma cells. Activation of the precursor, interaction with other matrix metalloproteinases and enzymic properties. *J. Biol. Chem.* 1995; 270: 6691-6697.

[384] Saitoh Y, Yanai H, Higaki S et al. Relationship between matrix metalloproteinase-7 and pit pattern in early stage colorectal cancer. *Gastrointest Endosc.* 2004; 59: 385-392.

[385] Zeng ZS, Guillem JG. Colocalisation of matrix metalloproteinase-9-mRNA and protein in human colorectal cancer stromal cells. *Br. J. Cancer.* 1996; 74: 1161-1167.

[386] Curran S, Dundas SR, Buxton J et al. Matrix metalloproteinase/tissue inhibitors of matrix metalloproteinase phenotype identifies poor prognosis colorectal cancers. *Clin. Cancer Res.* 2004; 10: 8229-8234.

[387] Roeb E, Arndt M, Jansen B et al. Simultaneous determination of matrix metalloproteinase (MMP)-7, MMP-1, -3, and -13 gene expression by multiplex PCR in colorectal carcinomas. *Int. J. Colorectal. Dis.* 2004; 19: 518-524.

[388] Gustavson MD, Crawford HC, Fingleton B, Matrisian LM. Tcf binding sequence and position determines beta-catenin and Lef-1 responsiveness of MMP-7 promoters. *Mol. Carcinog.* 2004; 41: 125-139.

[389] Ougolkov AV, Yamashita K, Mai M, Minamoto T. Oncogenic beta-catenin and MMP-7 (matrilysin) cosegregate in late-stage clinical colon cancer. *Gastroenterology.* 2002; 122: 60-71.

[390] Macfarlane SR, Seatter MJ, Kanke T et al. Proteinase-activated receptors. *Pharmacol. Rev* .2001; 53: 245-282.

[391] Bohm SK, McConalogue K, Kong W, Bunnett NW. Proteinase-Activated Receptors: New Functions for Old Enzymes. *News Physiol. Sci.* 1998; 13: 231-240.

[392] Kanke T, Takizawa T, Kabeya M, Kawabata A. Physiology and pathophysiology of proteinase-activated receptors (PARs): PAR-2 as a potential therapeutic target. *J. Pharmacol. Sci.* 2005; 97: 38-42.

[393] Hollenberg MD. Physiology and pathophysiology of proteinase-activated receptors (PARs): proteinases as hormone-like signal messengers: PARs and more. *J. Pharmacol. Sci.* 2005; 97: 8-13.

[394] D'Andrea MR, Derian CK, Leturcq D et al. Characterization of protease-activated receptor-2 immunoreactivity in normal human tissues. *J. Histochem. Cytochem.* 1998; 46: 157-164.

[395] Kunzelmann K, Schreiber R, Konig J, Mall M. Ion transport induced by proteinase-activated receptors (PAR2) in colon and airways. *Cell Biochem. Biophys.* 2002; 36: 209-214.

[396] Mall M, Gonska T, Thomas J et al. Activation of ion secretion via proteinase-activated receptor-2 in human colon. *Am. J. Physiol. Gastrointest. Liver Physiol.* 2002; 282: G200-210.

[397] Ohta T, Shimizu K, Yi S et al. Protease-activated receptor-2 expression and the role of trypsin in cell proliferation in human pancreatic cancers. *Int. J. Oncol.* 2003; 23: 61-66.

[398] Cottrell GS, Amadesi S, Grady EF, Bunnett NW. Trypsin IV, a novel agonist of protease-activated receptors 2 and 4. *J. Biol. Chem.* 2004; 279: 13532-13539.

[399] Darmoul D, Marie JC, Devaud H et al. Initiation of human colon cancer cell proliferation by trypsin acting at protease-activated receptor-2. *Br. J. Cancer.* 2001; 85: 772-779.

[400] Shi X, Gangadharan B, Brass LF et al. Protease-activated receptors (PAR1 and PAR2) contribute to tumor cell motility and metastasis. *Mol. Cancer Res.* 2004; 2: 395-402.

[401] Hjortoe GM, Petersen LC, Albrektsen T et al. Tissue factor-factor VIIa-specific up-regulation of IL-8 expression in MDA-MB-231 cells is mediated by PAR-2 and results in increased cell migration. *Blood.* 2004; 103: 3029-3037.

[402] Lynch CC, Crawford HC, Matrisian LM, McDonnell S. Epidermal growth factor upregulates matrix metalloproteinase-7 expression through activation of PEA3 transcription factors. *Int. J. Oncol.* 2004; 24: 1565-1572.

[403] Mimori K, Yamashita K, Ohta M et al. Coexpression of matrix metalloproteinase-7 (MMP-7) and epidermal growth factor (EGF) receptor in colorectal cancer: an EGF receptor tyrosine kinase inhibitor is effective against MMP-7-expressing cancer cells. *Clin. Cancer Res.* 2004; 10: 8243-8249.

[404] Shimamoto R, Sawada T, Uchima Y et al. A role for protease-activated receptor-2 in pancreatic cancer cell proliferation. *Int. J. Oncol.* 2004; 24: 1401-1406.

[405] D'Andrea MR, Derian CK, Santulli RJ, Andrade-Gordon P. Differential expression of protease-activated receptors-1 and -2 in stromal fibroblasts of normal, benign, and malignant human tissues. *Am. J. Pathol.* 2001; 158: 2031-2041.

[406] Gruber BL, Marchese MJ, Santiago-Schwarz F et al. Protease-activated receptor-2 (PAR-2) expression in human fibroblasts is regulated by growth factors and extracellular matrix. *J. Invest. Dermatol.* 2004; 123: 832-839.

[407] Kong W, McConalogue K, Khitin LM et al. Luminal trypsin may regulate enterocytes through proteinase-activated receptor 2. *Proc. Natl. Acad. Sci. U. S. A.* 1997; 94: 8884-8889.

[408] Cianchi F, Cortesini C, Fantappie O et al. Cyclooxygenase-2 activation mediates the proangiogenic effect of nitric oxide in colorectal cancer. *Clin Cancer Res.* 2004; 10: 2694-2704.

[409] Wagenaar-Miller RA, Hanley G, Shattuck-Brandt R et al. Cooperative effects of matrix metalloproteinase and cyclooxygenase-2 inhibition on intestinal adenoma reduction. *Br. J. Cancer.* 2003; 88: 1445-1452.

[410] Pai R, Nakamura T, Moon WS, Tarnawski AS. Prostaglandins promote colon cancer cell invasion; signaling by cross-talk between two distinct growth factor receptors. *Faseb. J.* 2003; 17: 1640-1647.

INDEX

A

aberrant methylation, 46
access, 18
accuracy, 31
acid, 17, 38, 49, 50, 63, 87
activated receptors, 61, 93, 96, 97, 98
activation, 35, 49, 52, 53, 55, 56, 60, 61, 62, 63, 88, 89, 90, 91, 93, 95, 96, 97, 98
addiction, 83
adenine, 33
adenocarcinoma(s), 11, 55, 57, 69, 77, 78, 86, 88, 94
adenoma(s), vii, 1, 3, 4, 5, 8, 12, 21, 23, 24, 25, 28, 29, 30, 31, 47, 48, 49, 51, 59, 60, 61, 64, 65, 69, 70, 71, 76, 77, 79, 85, 86, 87, 88, 98
adenosine, 34
adhesion, 90, 93
adolescence, 8, 11
age, 3, 8, 9, 11, 12, 14, 19, 29, 47
agent, 87
agonist, 63, 97
air, 27
airways, 97
algorithm, 71
alkaline, 55
allele, 33
alpha, 87
alpha1-antitrypsin, 94

alternative, 3, 45, 64, 69
amino, 38, 55, 61
amino acid(s), 38, 55
Amsterdam, 9, 10, 11, 12
amyloid precursor protein, 91
aneuploid, 39
angiogenesis, 3, 15, 53, 72, 93
angiogenic, 17, 90, 91
anhydrase, 22
animal models, 31, 49
anticancer, 86
antigen, 22, 58, 85, 94
anti-inflammatory drugs, 29, 51, 86, 88
antitumor, 17
APC, vii, 3, 4, 10, 11, 12, 22, 31, 35, 36, 37, 49, 52, 60, 69, 71, 76, 87
apoptosis, vii, 3, 31, 35, 39, 53, 68, 72, 79, 80, 81, 85, 90, 93
apoptotic, 53, 62, 90
arachidonic acid, 17, 50, 63
arginine, 55
artery, 61
Asian, 21
aspartate, 38
aspirin, 29, 86
assessment, 29, 46
asymptomatic, 20, 21, 23, 74
atherosclerosis, 55
attention, 17, 21, 49
atypical, 8, 47
autosomal dominant, 8, 13

B

autosomal recessive, 12
awareness, vii, 1

bacterial, 19
basal cell nevus syndrome, 13
base pair, 42
batimastat, 62
Bax, 80
B-cell, 36
Bcl-2, 4, 35, 36, 37, 53, 72, 80, 90
benign, 21, 25, 28, 70, 98
beta, 76, 79, 80, 89, 96
bias, 20
bile duct, 55
binding, 50, 62, 91, 96
biochemical, 22
biologic, 16
biological, 36, 61, 62, 65, 68, 89
biology, 29, 40, 75, 88
biomarker(s), 23, 29, 30, 31, 46, 77, 79
biopsy, 28
bipolar, 93
births, 11
bleeding, 27
blood, 16, 21, 55, 63, 74, 75
blood flow, 63
blood pressure, 55
blood vessels, 16
bonds, 55
bowel, 1, 8, 9, 11, 13, 14, 17, 18, 19, 21, 23, 29, 46, 65, 72, 73, 74, 75, 89
brain, 55, 91
breakdown, 56
breast, 13, 14, 35, 87, 90
breast cancer, 35, 87, 90
budding, 95
bypass, 22

C

cadherin, 22
cAMP, 50, 53

cancer(s), vii, viii, 1, 4, 7, 8, 9, 11, 12, 13, 14, 18, 19, 20, 21, 22, 28, 29, 30, 31, 35, 36, 37, 39, 40, 41, 42, 45, 46, 47, 49, 52, 55, 56, 57, 58, 59, 60, 61, 62, 63, 64, 65, 67, 68, 69, 70, 71, 72, 73, 74, 75, 76, 77, 78, 79, 80, 81, 82, 83, 84, 85, 86, 87, 88, 89, 90, 91, 92, 93, 94, 95, 96, 97, 98
cancer cells, 45, 56, 57, 60, 62, 69, 72, 80, 88, 90, 92, 93, 94, 96, 97
cancer progression, 58, 61, 90, 94
cancer screening, 9, 74, 75
cancer stem cells, 83
candidates, 30
capillary, 27
carboxyl groups, 55
carcinoembryonic antigen (CEA), 22, 94
carcinogen, 22
carcinogenesis, 1, 3, 4, 21, 22, 25, 31, 35, 42, 49, 51, 73, 75, 80, 81, 83, 87, 88, 93
carcinogenic pathway, 17, 19, 85
carcinoma, vii, 1, 3, 4, 21, 24, 29, 47, 48, 49, 51, 59, 60, 61, 65, 68, 69, 70, 72, 75, 76, 78, 81, 82, 84, 85, 86, 89, 92, 93, 95, 96
caspase, 53, 80
catheter, 27
cDNA, 41, 91
cell, viii, 4, 13, 15, 16, 17, 19, 31, 35, 36, 37, 38, 39, 42, 45, 49, 50, 52, 53, 57, 61, 62, 63, 73, 80, 81, 84, 87, 89, 91, 92, 93, 94, 95, 97, 98
cell cycle, 31, 53
cell growth, 39, 52, 62, 87, 89
cell invasion, 98
cell line(s), 42, 57, 61, 63, 80, 84, 91, 92, 95
cell membranes, 17
cell surface, 17, 61
cellular adhesion, 90
certainty, 30
cervical, 13, 79
chemical, 15
chemokines, 16, 17
chemoprevention, 79, 86, 90
chemopreventive agents, 31
chemotherapy, 39, 40, 65, 68
childhood, 13

cholangiocarcinoma, 20, 53, 90
cholangitis, 18, 19, 73
cholestasis, 19
chromatin, 45, 46
chromoendoscopy, 27, 28
chromosomal abnormalities, 35, 45
chromosomal instability (CIN), vii, 1, 5, 19, 35, 39, 40, 42, 65, 67, 69, 79
chromosome (s), 3, 8, 10, 12, 13, 82, 83, 86
classification, vii, 21, 23, 24, 28, 47, 69, 76, 78
cleavage, 61, 63
clinical, viii, 1, 3, 8, 10, 15, 20, 29, 37, 41, 47, 65, 67, 68, 70, 73, 75, 84, 86, 96
clinician(s), vii, 36
clones, 18
clustering, 8
c-myc, 52
coagulation, 55, 93
coding, 35
codon, 38
cohort, 18, 39
colectomy, 9, 14
colitis, 18, 19, 20, 50, 72, 73, 74
collagen, 15, 56, 93
colon cancer, 7, 8, 9, 11, 12, 18, 30, 31, 46, 52, 62, 63, 68, 70, 72, 74, 75, 76, 79, 80, 83, 84, 86, 87, 88, 89, 90, 93, 94, 96, 97, 98
colon carcinogenesis, 81, 87
colon polyps, 46
colonization, 19
colonoscopy, 20, 21, 22, 23, 77
colorectal, vii, viii, 1, 3, 4, 7, 8, 18, 19, 20, 21, 22, 23, 25, 27, 28, 29, 31, 36, 37, 39, 40, 42, 46, 47, 48, 49, 57, 58, 60, 61, 64, 65, 67, 68, 69, 70, 71, 72, 73, 74, 75, 76, 77, 79, 80, 81, 82, 83, 84, 85, 86, 87, 88, 89, 90, 92, 93, 94, 95, 96, 97, 98
colorectal adenocarcinoma, 69, 94
colorectal cancer (CRC), vii, viii, 1, 3, 4, 5, 7, 8, 9, 18, 11, 12, 13, 14, 17, 19, 20, 21, 22, 28, 29, 31, 33, 34, 35, 36, 37, 39, 40, 41, 42, 43, 46, 47, 49, 50, 52, 54, 56, 57, 58, 59, 61, 62, 63, 64, 65, 67, 68, 69, 70, 71, 72, 73, 74, 75, 76, 77, 79, 80, 81, 82, 83, 84, 85, 87, 88, 89, 90, 92, 93, 94, 95, 96, 97, 98
colorectum, vii, 22, 47, 48, 83, 85
complexity, 47
components, 25
conditioning, 89
connective tissue, 15, 17
consensus, 22, 78
continuing, 73
control, 17, 37, 53, 55, 75, 88, 90
conversion, 59, 96
correlation(s), 41, 76
cost-effective, 20, 41, 71
costs, 41
coverage, viii
COX-1, 50
COX-2, 17, 22, 49, 50, 51, 53, 63, 64, 72, 87, 90
COX-2 inhibitors, 49, 51, 53, 64
CpG islands, 45, 88
craniofacial, 14
crosstalk, 53, 98
culture, 62, 91
cyclin D1, 52, 89
cyclooxygenase, 22, 51, 63, 72, 86, 87, 88, 89, 90, 93, 98
cyclooxygenase-2, 63, 72, 86, 87, 88, 89, 90, 93, 98
cyclooxygenases, viii
cytochrome, 53, 90
cytokeratins, 86
cytokine(s), 16, 17, 50, 74
cytoplasm, 57
cytoprotective, 50
cytosine, 33, 45
cytotoxic, 18, 38, 81
cytotoxicity, 80

D

de novo, 1, 21, 25, 47, 75
death, 11, 20, 90
decay, 50
decoding, 71
defects, 22, 30, 33, 41

deficiency, 46, 69, 82
definition, 21, 23
deformation, 27
degradation, 52, 53, 92
degree, 21, 25, 30, 59
demand, 41
demographic data, 29
Denmark, 73
depressed, 24, 25, 27, 28, 77
derivatives, 58
destruction, 16
detection, 2, 22, 27, 28, 29, 30, 31, 41, 46, 71, 79, 82, 83
diabetes, 91
diagnostic, 1, 10, 41, 76
dietary, 29
differentiation, 37, 40
digestion, 55
dinucleotides, 42, 45
diploid, 39
disease progression, 78
diseases, 45
disorder, 10
distal, 12, 13, 18, 22, 74
distribution, 7, 22, 39, 42, 51
diversity, 50
division, 25
DNA, vii, 3, 5, 17, 19, 29, 33, 34, 36, 38, 41, 42, 45, 46, 47, 53, 69, 70, 75, 82, 83, 84, 85
DNA damage, 53
DNA repair, vii, 42, 47, 53
Drosophila, 4, 36, 37
drugs, 18, 29, 86, 88
duodenum, 55, 91
duration, 18
dysplasia, 19, 21, 74

E

E-cadherin, 22
eicosanoid(s), 17, 88, 89
elaboration, 61
elastin, 15
electrophoresis, 41
embryonic, 58, 67

encoding, 91
endocrine, 13
endometrial carcinoma, 78
endometrial hyperplasia, 78
endoscopic, vii, 1, 27, 28, 29, 65, 77, 78, 85
endoscopy, 13, 28, 77
endothelial cell(s), 16
endothelium, 61
English, 77
environment, 56, 60
environmental, 29, 50
enzyme(s), 15, 17, 33, 34, 50, 55, 56, 61, 63, 73, 89
epidemiological, 29, 49
epidermal growth factor receptor (EGFR), 53, 62, 63, 90, 94
epigenetic, vii, viii, 1, 4, 5, 22, 33, 45, 46, 47, 50, 65, 81, 83, 84
epigenetic alterations, 22, 45, 46
epigenetic mechanism, vii, viii, 1, 45
epigenetic silencing, vii, 4, 5, 33, 47
epithelial cells, 51, 53, 55, 78, 87, 88, 89, 90, 91
epithelial transport, 63
epithelium, 49, 50, 63, 96
ERK1, 62, 63
esophagus, 13, 14, 55, 78
etiology, 29, 31
Europe, 11
European, 74, 75
evidence, 1, 17, 19, 20, 23, 29, 30, 41, 47, 56, 61, 63, 94, 95
evolution, vii, 3, 47, 49
excision, 12, 19, 73
exposure, 29, 61
extracellular, viii, 15, 16, 56, 63, 91, 92, 98
extracellular matrix (ECM), viii, 16, 91, 92, 98

F

factor VII, 97
faecal, 21, 74
familial, 7, 71, 75, 76, 77, 81, 82, 86
familial polyposis coli, 77

family, 8, 12, 16, 29, 53, 61, 71
family history, 12, 29, 71
fecal, 74, 75
feces, 29
fibrinolysis, 55
fibroblasts, 63, 98
fibronectin, 15
fibrosarcoma, 92
fibrosis, 16, 19
fish, 49
fixation, 41
flora, 18
flow, 63
food, 55
forceps, 28
frameshift mutation, 5, 35, 38, 80

G

G protein, 52
gastric, 8, 9, 14, 35, 58, 60, 61, 92
gastritis, 78
gastrointestinal, 8, 11, 13, 14, 17, 22, 29, 56, 61, 73, 74, 76, 79, 82, 87, 88, 89, 94
gastrointestinal tract, 13, 14, 56, 61, 87, 88
gelatinase A, 92
gene(s), vii, 3, 4, 7, 8, 9, 10, 11, 12, 13, 14, 17, 19, 31, 33, 34, 35, 36, 37, 39, 40, 41, 42, 45, 46, 47, 49, 51, 52, 69, 71, 74, 79, 80, 81, 82, 83, 86, 87, 88, 94, 96
gene expression, 45, 81, 88, 96
gene silencing, 46, 83
generation, 17, 72
genetic(s), viii, 3, 4, 5, 7, 8, 18, 19, 21, 29, 31, 34, 35, 39, 40, 41, 45, 46, 47, 48, 49, 65, 68, 69, 70, 73, 76, 78
genetic abnormalities, 45
genetic alteration, 3, 4, 19, 21, 29, 31, 46
genetic defect, 30, 41
genetic instability, 4, 39, 47, 69, 73
genetic screening, 31
genetic syndromes, 29
genetic testing, 31
genome, 4, 34, 46
genomic, 42, 70

germ line, 33
germline mutations, 3
gland, 68
glycine, 38
glycogen synthase kinase, 52, 89
glycoproteins, 15
goblet cells, 91
G-protein, 61
granulomas, 18
groups, 55, 59
growth, 3, 4, 15, 16, 17, 23, 35, 36, 37, 39, 52, 53, 60, 61, 62, 63, 72, 76, 80, 85, 86, 87, 89, 90, 97, 98
growth factor (s), 4, 16, 17, 35, 36, 37, 53, 62, 76, 80, 97, 98
GSK-3, 52, 53
guanine, 34, 45
guidelines, 20, 41, 47, 71, 82
gut, 74

H

head, 24
healing, 17, 61, 72
health, 74
heterogeneity, 41, 69
heterogeneous, 1, 16, 47
heterotrimeric, 52
heterozygosity, 4, 5, 22, 71, 76
high-frequency, 42, 79, 81, 82
high-risk, 31
histidine, 38
histogenesis, 48
histological, 19, 22, 85
histology, 19, 31, 47
histone, 45
histopathology, 75, 82
homeostasis, 15
hormone(s), 50, 96
host, 15, 16
human (s), 4, 22, 31, 33, 42, 53, 55, 56, 60, 68, 69, 72, 76, 80, 83, 87, 88, 89, 90, 91, 92, 93, 94, 95, 96, 97, 98
human brain, 91
hypermethylation, 19, 40, 42, 46, 81, 84

hyperplasia, 78
hyperplastic polyps, viii, 28, 47
hypertrophy, 89
hypomethylation, 50
hypotension, 61

I

identification, 7, 22, 31, 46, 71, 82
IGF-I, 4
IL-8, 97
ileum, 18
illumination, 63
image analysis, 31
imaging, 1, 28
imbalances, 68
immune response, 18, 39
immunogenicity, 80
immunohistochemical, 57, 92
immunohistochemistry, 31, 57, 71
immunoreactivity, 56, 57, 91, 94, 97
immunotherapy, 84
in situ, 24
in vivo, 22, 80, 93, 95
incidence, 18, 22, 23, 29, 30, 31, 40, 47, 77
inclusion, 1, 31, 48
indicators, 46
indigenous, 18
induction, 18, 59, 63, 72, 90
inflammation, viii, 15, 17, 19, 38, 50, 55, 63, 71, 72, 73, 74
inflammatory, 1, 15, 16, 17, 18, 19, 28, 38, 40, 50, 72, 73, 74, 89
inflammatory bowel disease (IBD), 1, 17, 18, 19, 20, 72, 73, 74, 89
inflammatory cells, 17, 19
inflammatory mediators, 16
inflammatory response(s), 15, 16, 18, 38
inhibition, vii, viii, 1, 49, 53, 58, 60, 64, 85, 87, 98
inhibitor(s), 11, 53, 55, 58, 62, 64, 84, 86, 87, 89, 92, 93, 94, 95, 96, 97
inhibitory, 52, 60, 63, 64
initiation, vii, 3, 11, 46, 59, 60, 76
injection, 28

injury, 15
innominate, 28
inositol, 63
insertion, 38, 41
instabilities, 22
instability, vii, 1, 4, 5, 8, 10, 19, 22, 31, 33, 34, 39, 41, 42, 46, 47, 60, 65, 67, 68, 69, 70, 71, 73, 79, 80, 81, 82, 83, 84, 85, 86
insulin-like growth factor I, 4
insults, 16
interaction(s), viii, 15, 37, 96
interactions
interferons, 16
interleukin(s), 16, 62
international, 22, 71
interpretation, 41, 79
interval, 18, 30
intervention, vii, 7, 29, 30, 31, 49
intestinal tract, 72
intestine, 13, 14, 18, 55, 63, 77, 85
invasive cancer, 21, 29
invasive lesions, 28
isoforms, 50, 55, 57, 88
isoleucine, 38
isozymes, 88

J

Japanese, 21, 23, 76, 77

K

Ki-67, 85
kidney, 55
kinase(s), 13, 37, 52, 62, 63, 74, 87, 88, 97
King, 88

L

laminin, 15, 95
large intestine, 18, 85
latency, 18
late-stage, 96
lead, 19, 20, 22, 33, 39, 46

leiomyoma, 28
lesions, viii, 18, 21, 22, 23, 25, 27, 28, 29, 47, 65, 72, 77
leukemia, 36, 92
leukocyte(s), 15, 16, 17, 55, 91
leukotrienes, 17
lifetime, 3, 8, 34
ligand(s), 53, 61, 62, 63, 90
linear model, 3
links, 40, 73
lipid, 88, 89
lipoproteins, 17
literature, 41, 47, 68
liver, 55, 73, 80, 81, 95
liver metastases, 80, 81, 95
liver transplantation, 73
localization, 77, 80
location, 47, 86
loss of heterozygosity, 4, 5, 22
lumen, 55
lung, 13, 14, 35, 55, 56, 61, 92
lymph, 17, 25, 28, 39, 57
lymph node, 25, 28, 39, 57
lymphatic, 57
lymphocytes, 16, 17, 38, 81
lymphoid tissue, 18
lymphoma, 36
lysine, 55

M

macrophages, 16, 17, 53
malignancy, 7, 28, 48, 74
malignant, 15, 22, 24, 25, 35, 57, 70, 72, 92, 95, 96, 98
malignant cells, 25
malignant tumors, 70
mammogram, 13
management, 77
manifold, 56
matrix, viii, 1, 15, 16, 17, 56, 59, 73, 91, 92, 93, 94, 95, 96, 97, 98
matrix metalloproteinase, 1, 56, 59, 73, 93, 94, 95, 96, 97, 98
MCC, 22

Mcl-1, 53
measurement, 62
mediators, 15, 16, 87
MEK, 37
melanoma, 63
membranes, 17, 39, 61
memory, 17, 72
messenger RNA, 50
messengers, 96
meta-analysis, 68
metabolic, 17
metabolites, 17
metalloproteinase(s), 1, 56, 59, 62, 73, 92, 93, 94, 95, 96, 97, 98
metastases, 28, 80, 81, 95
metastasis, viii, 16, 39, 40, 56, 57, 59, 62, 63, 68, 72, 80, 93, 94, 95, 97
metastatic, viii, 11, 17, 39, 56, 57, 72, 86, 93
methionine, 38
methylation, vii, 22, 45, 46, 47, 69, 83, 84, 85, 88
MGMT, vii, 36, 42, 47, 85
mice, 19, 22, 42, 49, 71, 86, 87
microarray, 41, 79, 83
microbial, 15, 18
microcirculation, 17
microenvironment, 15, 16, 17, 50, 63, 65
microorganisms, 18
microsatellites, 5, 34, 35, 42
microscopy, 19
microsurgery, 28, 77, 78
migration, 16, 17, 62, 92, 95, 97
Minnesota, 74, 75
minority, 30
mitochondrial, 53, 90
mitogen-activated protein kinase (MAPK), 37, 53, 63, 94,
mitogenesis, 61
mitogenic, 62, 63
mitotic checkpoint, 90
MMP(s), 56, 57, 59, 60, 61, 62, 63, 64, 91, 93, 94, 95, 96, 97
MMP-2, 59, 93
MMP-3, 93, 95
MMP-9, 59, 91, 93

models, 22, 31, 49
modulation, 31, 50, 84
molecular biology, 75, 88
molecular markers, 46
molecular mechanisms, vii, viii, 1, 43
molecules, 15, 55, 56, 61
morbidity, 29
mortality, 28, 29, 75
mothers, 4, 36, 37
mouse model, 73, 76, 87, 93
mRNA, 50, 57, 58, 80, 88, 93
MSS, 5, 34, 42
mucin, 86
mucosa, vii, 13, 18, 19, 21, 22, 24, 25, 27, 28, 47, 56, 57, 58, 94
multidisciplinary, 49
multiplicity, 64
muscle, 61
mutant, 49, 87
mutation(s), vii, 3, 4, 5, 7, 8, 10, 11, 12, 13, 22, 29, 31, 33, 34, 35, 38, 39, 41, 42, 43, 45, 47, 49, 52, 60, 69, 71, 79, 80, 82, 91
mutation rate, 12

N

Nash, 82
natural, 12, 58
necrosis, 16, 90
neoangiogenesis, 17
neoplasia, vii, viii, 1, 13, 15, 17, 19, 21, 23, 24, 25, 27, 28, 29, 46, 48, 65, 67, 71, 74, 76, 77, 78, 79, 85, 86
neoplasm(s), 15, 18, 33, 46, 50, 78, 92
neoplastic, 3, 15, 17, 18, 21, 22, 24, 45, 46, 47, 79, 81, 94
neoplastic cells, 3, 15, 17, 18, 45
neoplastic tissue, 17
network, 17, 27
neurogenic, 73
neuronal cells, 55
neurons, 91
nevus, 13
NF-kB, 50, 53
nitric oxide, 22, 98

nitric oxide synthase (NOS), 22
nitrogen, 17, 19
nodes, 25
non-random, 70
non-steroidal anti-inflammatory drugs (NSAIDs), viii, 29, 49, 51
normal, 18, 19, 22, 25, 29, 31, 35, 38, 41, 45, 47, 50, 56, 57, 58, 83, 94, 97, 98
North America, 20
Norway, 67
nucleotide sequence, 5, 91
nucleotides, 33, 38

O

obligate, 29
occult blood, 21, 75
oncogene(s), 45, 80, 81, 90, 93
oncogenesis, 73
oral, 13
organization, 76
ovarian, 13, 14, 35, 92
ovarian cancer, 92
ovary(ies), 13, 56
oxidative damage, 12
oxidative stress, 19
oxide, 22, 73, 98
oxygen, 17, 19

P

p53, 3, 19, 22, 35, 40, 42, 53, 69, 79, 80, 85, 86, 90
pancreas, 13, 14, 61
pancreatic, 14, 55, 60, 63, 78, 91, 93, 94, 95, 97
pancreatic acinar cell, 55
pancreatic cancer, 14, 63, 78, 93, 94, 97
pancreatitis, 56, 91
paracrine, 50, 63
paradigm shift, 67
paraffin-embedded, 57
pathogenesis, 18, 22, 46, 71, 74
pathogenic, 20, 46

Index

pathology, 13
pathophysiological, 56
pathophysiology, 93, 96
pathways, vii, viii, 1, 3, 4, 5, 17, 19, 35, 37, 49, 51, 52, 53, 65, 67, 69, 76, 81, 87
patients, 1, 7, 8, 10, 11, 12, 13, 14, 17, 18, 19, 20, 28, 30, 32, 40, 41, 42, 50, 55, 56, 60, 64, 65, 67, 68, 69, 70, 71, 72, 73, 74, 76, 80, 81, 83, 85, 91, 94
PCR, 41, 57, 83, 96
penetrance, 8, 11, 12, 13
peptide, 55, 61, 63
peptide bonds, 55
phagocytosis, 17
pharmacological, 49
phenotype(s), 4, 12, 43, 46, 47, 57, 69, 70, 82, 84, 85, 92, 96
phosphorylates, 63
phosphorylation, 52, 53, 62, 63, 89, 94
physiology, 55
PI3K, 37, 52, 53
placebo, 86
play, 4, 7, 49, 55, 59, 60, 61, 64
politics, 74
polymerase, 33, 41, 57
polymorphisms, 74, 95
polyp(s), vii, viii, 8, 9, 11, 12, 13, 14, 22, 23, 24, 28, 30, 46, 47, 48, 50, 63, 71, 76, 77, 78, 85, 86, 89
polypectomy, 14, 28, 77
poor, 37, 40, 42, 56, 68, 95, 96
population, 3, 19, 20, 23, 30, 31, 35, 41, 72, 74, 75, 77, 79, 82
power, 27
preclinical, 86
prediction, 65
predictive accuracy, 31
predictive marker, 36
pressure, 55
prevention, vii, 2, 11, 28, 29, 31, 48, 64, 79, 87
primary tumor, 80, 95
probability, 30
proctitis, 18
production, 17, 50, 53, 55, 62

prognosis, 1, 20, 21, 24, 38, 40, 42, 46, 56, 60, 65, 68, 72, 85, 95, 96
prognostic marker, 1, 65, 93
program, 74
progressive, 45
proinflammatory, 17
proliferation, viii, 15, 16, 17, 52, 53, 59, 62, 68, 81, 85, 90, 93, 94, 97
promote, 98
promoter, vii, 35, 40, 45, 46, 50, 70, 73, 81, 84, 88, 95
promoter region, vii, 45, 46, 50, 84
prostaglandin(s), 17, 49, 50, 51, 54, 63, 72, 86, 87, 88, 89, 90, 91
prostanoids, 17
prostate, 13, 14, 35, 56, 92
prostate cancer, 13, 92
proteases, 61, 71, 91
protective mechanisms, 58
protein(s), 4, 15, 22, 34, 35, 36, 37, 38, 39, 41, 46, 50, 52, 53, 55, 56, 57, 58, 80, 82, 86, 88, 94, 96
proteinase, 56, 59, 61, 73, 92, 93, 96, 97, 98
proteoglycans, 15
proteolysis, 61
proteolytic enzyme, 56
proteomics, 81
protocols, 41
prototype, vii, 29
proximal, 12, 37, 47, 70, 79
puberty, 11
public health, 74

R

race, 29
radical, 29
random, 4, 46
range, 55
ras, 3, 22, 35, 42, 50, 69, 76, 79, 87
rat(s), 86, 87
reactant, 94
reactive oxygen, 15, 17
reactive oxygen species, 15
reactivity, 16

reading, 38
Receiver Operating Characteristics, 67
receptors, 1, 17, 51, 53, 61, 63, 89, 93, 96, 97, 98
recognition, 45, 70
rectum, 11, 14, 18, 22, 24
recurrence, 57, 78
reduction, 50, 64, 98
reflection, 43
regional, 25, 28
regression, 61
regulation, vii, 50, 53, 57, 61, 72, 83, 84, 88, 92, 97
regulators, 31
relationship, 25, 30, 43, 53, 79, 84, 96
relatives, 73
relaxation, 61
relevance, 75, 93
remodeling, 15, 83
renal, 8, 9
repair, vii, 3, 5, 8, 9, 12, 16, 19, 22, 33, 34, 35, 41, 42, 46, 47, 53, 69, 73, 82, 83
repair system, 33
replication, 8, 33, 34
repression, 45
research, viii, 10, 22, 23, 31, 40, 48, 65
researchers, 23
resection, 28, 77
residues, 45
resistance, 90
responsiveness, 96
retinoblastoma, 37
retinoic acid, 49, 87
reverse transcriptase, 31, 85
risk, vii, 3, 7, 8, 9, 11, 12, 13, 14, 17, 18, 20, 28, 29, 30, 31, 34, 46, 50, 56, 75, 76, 79, 85, 86
risk assessment, 46
risk factors, 19, 29, 30
RNA, 50, 57, 95
rodents, 19
rofecoxib, 86, 87

S

saline, 28
science, 74
search(es), 29, 31, 46
searching, 34, 46
secretion, 96, 97
segregation, 60
sensitivity, 41, 82
series, 57, 75
serine, 13, 37, 55, 56, 59, 61, 93
serum, 92
shares, 29, 30
sigmoidoscopy, 23, 75
signaling, 14, 35, 52, 53, 63, 72, 76, 80, 89, 98
signaling pathway, 52
signals, 3, 52, 53, 80
signs, 17
sites, 15, 55
skin, 55
small intestine, 13, 18, 55
smooth muscle, 61
solid tumors, 17, 84
somatic mutations, 4
species, 15, 17, 19
specificity, 41
specter, 51
sporadic, vii, 5, 7, 8, 11, 19, 30, 33, 40, 41, 46, 47, 52, 68, 72, 75, 76, 79, 81, 82, 84, 88
stability, 5, 50, 88
stages, viii, 47, 78
stem cells, 17, 83
steroids, 18
stomach, 14, 55, 56, 78
strategies, 20, 39
stratification, 65
strength, 30
stress, 19
stroma, viii, 17, 50, 56, 72, 93
stromal, 15, 17, 60, 96, 98
stromal cells, 17, 60, 96
stromal fibroblasts, 98
structural changes, 22
submucosa, 18, 21, 24, 25, 28
suppression, 45, 83

Index

suppressor, 3, 10, 12, 13, 34, 35, 45, 46, 84, 87, 90
surgery, 4, 29, 34, 35, 37, 38, 39, 67, 83
surgical, 14, 20, 28, 29, 75
surgical intervention, 29
surgical resection, 28
surveillance, 9, 11, 12, 20, 30, 74
survival, 15, 17, 20, 40, 46, 53, 67, 68, 69, 72, 84, 85, 95
Survivin, 53, 78
susceptibility, 20, 39, 46, 90
symptoms, 11
synchronous, 40
syndrome, vii, 1, 7, 10, 11, 12, 13, 52, 70, 71
synthesis, 17, 50, 51, 64
systems, vii, viii, 1, 16, 22, 51, 52, 54, 56, 61, 65

T

T cell(s), 4, 17, 18, 37, 39, 72, 80, 89
T lymphocytes, 81
tar, 28
targets, 63, 90
technology, 36
teens, 11
teeth, 85
TEM, 28
tetracyclines, 58, 92
TGF, 4, 14, 35, 36, 37, 38, 62, 80
theory, 21, 64
therapeutic, viii, 1, 41, 60, 65, 87, 96
therapy, 2, 36, 40, 46, 48, 51, 64, 65, 90
threonine, 13, 37, 38
thrombin, 61, 63
thymidine, 34
thyroid, 11, 13, 14
thyroid cancer, 11
TIA, 50, 88
time, 7, 14, 20, 21, 30, 74
timing, 36
TIMP, 93
TIMP-1, 93
tissue, 15, 17, 18, 28, 29, 31, 41, 57, 71, 82, 92, 95, 96

tissue homeostasis, 15
Tokyo, 91
toxicity, 87
Toyota, 84
transcription, 35, 37, 45, 46, 49, 51, 53, 89, 97
transcription factor, 37, 49, 97
transcription factors, 37, 97
transcriptional, 45, 88
transcripts, 57
transformation, 17, 35, 46
transformations, 22
transforming growth factor, 4, 35, 36, 37, 62, 80
transgenic, 49
transition, 25, 60
translation, 50
translocations, 5
transmembrane, 61
transplantation, 73
transport, 61, 63, 89, 97
trial, 86
triggers, 63
trypsin, 55, 56, 57, 58, 59, 61, 62, 63, 64, 91, 92, 93, 94, 97, 98
tubular, 28
tumor(s), viii, 3, 5, 8, 9, 10, 11, 12, 13, 15, 17, 18, 21, 23, 24, 28, 29, 31, 34, 35, 37, 39, 40, 41, 42, 45, 46, 47, 50, 56, 57, 58, 60, 61, 62, 63, 64, 65, 68, 69, 70, 72, 73, 75, 76, 77, 79, 80, 81, 82, 83, 84, 86, 87, 90, 91, 92, 93, 94, 95, 97
tumor cells, viii, 17, 56, 68, 69, 91, 95
tumor growth, 15
tumor invasion, 17, 40, 94, 95
tumor necrosis factor (TNF), 53, 90
tumor progression, 29
tumor proliferation, 81
tumorigenesis, 23, 68, 71, 73, 81, 85, 90
type 1 collagen, 56
tyrosine, 37, 38, 62, 97

U

ulcerative colitis, 17, 19, 50, 74
ultrasound, 13

uniform, 41

V

variability, 41
variable, 22
variance, 31
vascular, 53
VEGF, 53
vessels, 16, 17, 25
visible, 22

W

Washington, 72
Weinberg, 68
WHO classification, 21
withdrawal, 64
women, 37
World Health Organization (WHO), 21, 78
wound healing, 17, 61, 72

Y

yield, 41, 42